Thought for foo

Margaret Sumner

Thought for food

Oxford New York Toronto Melbourne
OXFORD UNIVERSITY PRESS
1981

Oxford University Press, Walton Street, Oxford OX2 6DP

London Glasgow New York Toronto
Delhi Bombay Calcutta Madras Karachi
Kuala Lumpur Singapore Hong Kong Tokyo
Nairobi Dar es Salaam Cape Town
Melbourne Wellington
and associate companies in
Beirut Berlin Ibadan Mexico City

British Library Cataloguing in Publication Data
Sumner, Margaret
Thought for food.
1. Nutrition
I. Title
612'.3   TX353   80–49863
ISBN   0–19–217690–0
ISBN   0–19–286003–8 Pbk

Set, printed and bound in Great Britain by
Cox & Wyman Ltd, Reading

Contents

Foreword

In an affluent society, there is plenty to eat. Most of us are interested in food: cooking it, growing it, reading about it, and eating it all give tremendous enjoyment to different people.

Recently, however, this joyous approach has been replaced with a seriousness about eating which threatens to ruin the whole process. We are constantly advised which foods are good or bad for us and, moreover, different experts frequently contradict each other. It is tempting to throw your hands in the air and ignore all the advice.

This is a pity, because you can improve your diet, and enjoy your food as well. I have written this book to help you to do that. I have tried to give the *reasons* for the current advice about diet, so that you can make your own mind up. If you just love lots of sugar in your tea, or are mad about new white bread with lashings of butter, have them! You can offset any risks involved if you know something about food, or you may even decide to take the risks if you know what they are.

I am indebted to many people who helped me, but I wish to thank four of them especially. Wilfred Agar first made me interested in the common sense of nutrition. Jean Battersby read the book and commented (politely in most cases but always helpfully!) on the parts that were not clear. Mark Wahlqvist made invaluable suggestions on some errors and particularly some omissions in an early draft. Finally, my husband John believed against all odds that I would finish; that it would be interesting; and then took the children swimming while I wrote it!

March 1980   Margaret Sumner

1 Quantity

The primary function of food is to provide energy. All food contains energy which has been trapped by plants from the sun and stored in chemical bonds: by breaking down the chemical bonds in food we obtain the energy to stay alive. Food has other functions too, but if the diet is a varied one and enough is eaten to satisfy energy requirements, these other functions will be covered.

Because energy supply is the primary function of food, I have started this book by describing *how much* food we eat, leaving the other functions of food until later. The balance between the quantity of food a man eats and the amount of work he does in staying alive is called 'energy balance' and is the subject of this first chapter. When the balance goes wrong, the status quo is not maintained: either he eats too much and gets fat; or he eats too little and starves. These situations are the subjects of the chapters which follow.

What are calories and joules?

The energy contained in any one food is related to how much heat is given off when that food is burnt. It is measured in the laboratory in the following way. A small quantity of food is placed inside a heavy metal vessel called a 'bomb calorimeter' which is sealed and immersed in water. The food is then ignited by means of electric wires and as the food burns the temperature of the water rises. The heat produced is measured in calories, one calorie being the amount of heat which raises the temperature of one gram of water by one degree.

The amounts of energy which concern nutritionists are larger than those usually dealt with by physicists, therefore the unit generally used in nutrition is the kilocalorie (kcal), which is 1,000 calories. By convention, Calorie spelt with a large 'C' has come to denote the kilocalorie, so when you see Calorie, that is the same as kilocalorie.

To make matters more complicated for the layman (and indeed many nutritionists!), another unit has now been introduced. That is the *joule*. It was introduced because it is a unit of energy, rather than a unit of heat like the calorie. Again, the kilojoule (1,000 joules) is used by nutritionists. The sign for a kilojoule is kJ. In this book, kilojoules (kJ) and kilocalories (kcal) are given throughout. If you are interested in nutrition, you will have to get used to thinking in kilojoules because in future the energy value of food will be expressed in these units rather than Calories.

Fats contain 38 kJ (9 kcal) of energy per gram, carbohydrates and proteins 20 kJ (4·5 kcal) per gram, and alcohol 30 kJ (7 kcal) per gram. To put it another way, to boil a kettle of water (2 pints) you would need the energy from 10 grams of butter, 22 grams of sugar, or one double scotch.

The bomb calorimeter experiment is simply an explosive imitation of the process which takes place when energy is obtained from food in the body. During metabolism the process is more controlled and takes place in several steps, but the end result is the same in terms of the total energy content of any one food: fats still produce 38 kJ per gram, carbohydrates and proteins 20 kJ per gram, and alcohol 30 kJ per gram.

How much energy do we need?

Half of the energy for living is spent on the basic processes which keep you alive, such as the heart beat, breathing, hormone synthesis, and the production of electrochemical gradients which produce nerve impulses. These basic processes continue whether you are asleep or awake and require a constant amount of energy from hour to hour and from day to day. In a normal adult, the amount used is about *4·2 kJ (1 kcal) every minute*. Nothing you do makes any difference to the amount of energy spent in this way, and about half the food you eat is used for it.

The other half of your food is used for the extra work done in addition to these basic processes, including all movement. As soon as you stand up, energy expenditure increases over the basic rate; walking increases it more, and running still more. Obviously this second component varies a great deal from moment to moment and from one person to another. For example, more food is needed for digging the garden than for watching television and a ballet dancer or a builder has an over-all need for more food than an office worker. Here are some examples of the requirements for various activities (these are additional to the basic requirements of 4·2 kJ per minute):

Activity	*Energy cost per minute*
Light housework	
Golf	
Walking (slowly)	10–20 kJ (2·5–5 kcal)
Bricklaying	
Driving a truck	
Walking (briskly)	
Jogging	20 30 kJ (5–7·5 kcal)
Tennis	
Cycling (not racing)	
Coal-mining	30–40 kJ (7·5–10 kcal)
Football	
Competitive swimming	
Hill climbing	over 40 kJ (10 kcal)
Lumberjacking	

These energy costs are calculated by measuring the amount of oxygen used while performing the various tasks, since it is the combination of food with oxygen which produces energy. Thus energy requirements for extra work can be calculated: walking for one hour at 6 kilometres (4 m.) per hour uses 1,250 kJ (300 kcal) (three pints of beer or one 50–gram chocolate bar, for the diet conscious!).

What is energy balance?

The process of turning food into energy is complex. However, it is well understood and there is nothing magical about it; it obeys the normal laws of conservation of energy. If the food you eat is just enough to provide for your personal energy expenditure then you are in 'energy balance' and your weight stays constant. If you eat too little, you burn up your own body tissues for energy, and starvation occurs. If you eat too much, you store the excess and you get fat.

The individual cannot consciously work out his own energy balance. For one thing, it is highly unlikely outside the laboratory that the total energy in food can be estimated with an accuracy greater than 10 to 20 per cent. The reasons for this are faulty memory about what was eaten, inaccurate weighing, and the uncertain composition of food (such variations as fat content of meat, sugar content of fruit, even the generosity of your host as he pours the whisky are unknown factors). It is equally difficult to work out accurately how much energy is being used: the basic requirements can be calculated, but the extra allowance for work varies from minute to minute and is impossible to estimate accurately. Unconscious regulation is much more effective (see page 5). However, knowledge about energy balance has some use for the individual if his weight begins to alter, because it allows him to choose high- or low-energy foods, or make some adjustments to his activity level.

The people who must have detailed information about energy balance, and who use it to great effect, are those responsible for planning a diet for a group of people over an extended period in places like boarding schools, army barracks, prisons, and holiday camps. Sometimes diet has to be planned for the whole nation. For example, in 1939 it was necessary to make plans to feed 45 million people in Britain for an indefinite period of war with limited imports. Nutritionists and agriculturalists together worked out how many kilojoules (Calories in those days!) were needed, and how they could be produced most effectively. By a marvellous combination of knowledge and skill, and helped by a judicious use of propaganda, the diet of the nation was actually improved over the war years, and no one starved. Contrast this to the German experience in 1914 when the great German nutritionist, Rubner, advised the government that a high intake of meat was necessary to build strong men, and land was left for grazing cattle and sheep instead of being turned over to grain production. Since an acre of land produces six times as much food-energy when used for growing grain as it does when used for grazing, total food-energy production was considerably reduced and in the late years of the war when

Germany imported no food many civilians tragically starved. Hence it has been said that a nutritionist was as much to blame as any German general for losing the war.

Is energy balance regulated?

Most people eat enough food for the work they do and their body weight stays fairly constant. Consider the average man weighing 75 kilograms (165 lb) at 20 years of age. During the next forty years his daily energy expenditure will vary widely from a rate that is almost basal (the time he went in for cross-country skiing and broke both legs and lay for six weeks in plaster), to three or four times that rate (the time he went in for cross-country skiing and did not break his legs!). To provide energy over forty years to suit these varying needs he will eat approximately 20 tons of food (160 million kJ or 40 million kcal), and his food intake will be matched day by day to his energy requirements. An *error of only 1 per cent* in the control system would mean an excess or deficit of nearly 2 million kJ (half a million kcal). If this were excess, instead of weighing 75 kilograms at 60 years of age, he would weigh 119 kilograms (270 lb); if it were deficit, he would die. Clearly, since most people neither weigh 119 kilograms at 60 years of age nor die of starvation, food intake is matched to energy expenditure with a degree of accuracy which is better than 1 per cent.

The accuracy of the regulating system is remarkable in the face of the great changes in weight which result from extremely small excesses in daily food intake. A weight gain of 8 kilograms (16 lb) between the ages of 20 and 40 would be produced by eating an excess of 42 kJ (10 kcal) per day, that is half a teaspoonful of sugar or a piece of butter the size of a large pea! The same applies to changes in physical activity if they go on for a long time. For example, if you change from a manual to an automatic gear change in your car, the reduction in work necessary to drive could result in a weight gain of several kilograms over the period of your driving life.

What is the mechanism that matches the amount of food so accurately to our energy needs? This remains one of the principal unanswered questions of nutrition. It is known that there are centres in the brain that produce eating behaviour; thus if a certain part of the brain is stimulated in a rat, the animal will eat and eat and go on eating until it becomes too fat to move. Conversely, there are other brain centres which, when stimulated, will produce the opposite effect: the animal abstains totally from eating and will die unless forcibly fed. What is still unknown is what factors influence these centres, what turns them off and on; that is, what makes you start eating, and what makes you stop. However, although we remain ignorant of the mechanisms, it is indisputable that the quantity of food is altered according to the energy expenditure in normal circumstances, and weight stays fairly constant once adulthood is reached.

What has gone wrong?

In a typical affluent society there are indications that this well-regulated system may be breaking down. A study carried out by the Metropolitan Life Insurance Company in 1960 in the United States showed an increasing tendency for people to gain weight as they grew older. The average gain for a woman was 10 kilograms (22 lb) between the ages of 20 and 60 years. This gain was spread over the whole period; there was no such thing as a 'middle-age spread', the process started at 20! Thus in our society today obesity has become a problem, and it is pertinent to ask what has gone wrong with the regulating system.

To put on weight you need *at some stage to eat food in excess of your energy requirements*. Therefore the question we are asking is: do fat people eat more, or do they spend less energy? To answer this, let's look at food first, then at energy expenditure.

When it comes to eating, humans behave differently from other animals. Animals in their natural state search for food when they are hungry. This behaviour seems to result in good control of body weight; it is very rare to find an obese animal.

Man in an affluent society behaves differently. He is surrounded by food and he never has to hunt for it. His eating behaviour therefore tends to be dictated by habit rather than hunger; three (or four) meals a day is part of the pattern of modern life. In addition, business lunches, a drink after work, a beer with the boys, passing the chocolates in front of the television, coffee mornings with the neighbours: these endless social occasions are part of our daily life, and each one is accompanied by food. The normal signals are ignored, making the regulating system ineffective. On the eating side of the equation, therefore, we are ruled by habit and social custom, rather than need.

Now let's look at activity. Does our activity level control our food intake? An experiment by Jean Mayer, a leading American nutritionist, may have some bearing on the problem. He divided some rats into small groups and made each group run around on a treadmill for varying periods of time: the first group for one hour a day, the second for two hours, and so on. He gave all the animals free access to food and he found that for most groups the rats doing more exercise ate more food. In other words, food intake was being matched to energy output, and the body weight stayed constant. However, in those rats doing very little exercise and confined to their cages for most of the day, food intake was not reduced enough and they became fat.

Can a parallel be drawn between these fat rats and man in modern society? Jean Mayer measured the food consumption of men at various levels of energy expenditure. He found that the men behaved like the rats. Men in occupations requiring high expenditure of energy regulated their food intake accordingly. But men at the bottom of the range, in sedentary jobs, regulated poorly, and ate too much.

Our lives today, in contrast to those of our ancestors, are very inactive: we drive rather than walk, we work at desks rather than in the fields, we sit sometimes for a whole evening watching television. Modern man may represent the rat that is only on the treadmill for one hour each day, his energy expenditure is very low and he is not reducing his food intake to match it. He is in positive energy balance; that is, he is eating more than he needs, and he will gain weight.

Does this mean that fat people are fat because they are below a critical activity level? Differences of this kind could explain why some people are fat and others are thin, just as easily as differences in the amount of food eaten. Scientists looking for differences in activity levels have made some interesting observations. Time-lapse photographs were taken of children playing in a swimming pool over a fifteen-minute period. When the film was viewed, it was clear that some children jumped and splashed and moved around constantly, while others tended to stand still and watch. Similar observations were made on children playing basketball: some jumped up and down and ran around while waiting for the ball, whereas others tended to stand still and wait for the ball to come to them. When the children were weighed, it was found that there was a much higher proportion of fat children in the inactive group, while the active children tended to be thin. The point to stress here is that all the children were ostensibly engaged in the *same* physical activity, but some were spending far more energy than others.

There are all sorts of ways in which so-called active people spend extra energy; they may jiggle and jump around like the children in the experiment; they may sleep for shorter periods and even when asleep they may toss around a lot; they may sit with many of their muscles tensed while their plump friends relax like a jelly. Spending, say, an extra 40 kJ (10 kcal) per hour like this would add up to a weight loss of 160 grams (over a quarter of a pound) in one week. In other words, an 'active' and an 'inactive' person, starting at the same weight, could eat exactly the same food and ostensibly indulge in the same level of physical activity, and in one year the 'inactive' one would be 8 kilograms (16 lb) heavier than the other.

It has been established that fat people tend to eat less, not more, than thin people, so possibly the main difference between fat and thin people is related to the activity level rather than to food intake. Such differences may turn out to be all-important in determining whether you are fat or not. The genetically inactive person would be at an advantage in a situation where food is short, such as a primitive food-hunting society, and natural selection may have meant that more of these people have survived. In the present affluent society with food all around us, such people will get fat. The next two chapters describe the problem of overweight.

2 What is obesity?

They would sit down at lunchtime to a table set with three geese, browned to perfection, deliciously garnished with running gravy, green peas and new potatoes veined with dark sprigs of mint, baked onions, asparagus, roast potatoes, Yorkshire pudding and broad beans in parsley sauce . . . A typical breakfast was three eggs, four six inch rashers of home cured bacon, three very thick brown sausages and a slice of fried bread.

H. E. Bates, *The Darling Buds of May* (1935)

Ma Larkins, who prepared the meals described above, was fat. She knew she was fat and she liked being fat. She took a great joy in cooking for herself and her family, accepting food as a heaven-sent gift to be enjoyed until you could eat no more. I have put her at the head of this chapter to maintain a sense of proportion. 'Thin is in, stout is out' is the catch-phrase of today; fat people are regarded as gluttons or sloths or both and an increasing number of experts urge us to stay thin and be healthy. To help understand the wide diversity of expert opinion, I have tried in this chapter to answer three questions. Are you fat? How does it happen? Is it wrong to be fat? In the chapter that follows, I have discussed what you can do about it. Select the bits that interest you most. But remember Ma Larkins and those roast geese, and don't take any of it so seriously that you stop enjoying your food altogether.

Are you fat?

Ma Larkins knew she was fat, but if you do not have quite her ample proportions, have forgotten what size you were when you were 18, and have no honest friends, how are you to know if you are fat? Here are six simple tests which will give you a quick answer:

1. Lie on your back on the floor and place a ruler with one end on the lower end of your breast bone and the other end on your pubic bone. If the ruler touches the skin on your tummy, you are probably fat. (If, as one of my fat friends complained, you put one end of the ruler on your chest and the other end points to the ceiling, you are certainly fat, unless, of course, you are pregnant.)

2. Subtract your waist measurement in centimetres or inches from your height; if the answer is less than 90 centimetres (36 in.) you are probably fat.

3. If your waist measurement is more than your chest measurement, you are probably fat.

4. Calculate an acceptable weight for your height as follows: allow 45 kilograms (100 lb) for the first 150 centimetres (60 in.) of your height and add 2·2 kilograms (5 lb) for every extra 2·5 centimetres (1 in.) if you are a woman; the figures for men are 48 kilograms (106 lb) for the first 150 centimetres and 2·7 kilograms (6 lb) for every extra 2·5 centimetres. If your actual weight exceeds the calculated total, you are probably fat.

5. Sit on a chair without your clothes on and lean slightly forward. Now pick up a fold of skin between your navel and your hip bone, parallel to your groin. If the fold of skin is thicker than two fingers, you are probably fat.

6. Lastly, and the best test of all, take off all your clothes and stand in front of a mirror. Does anywhere bulge? Reach your arms in the air; you should be able to see your ribs well enough to count them. Jump up and down; do you wobble? (You must allow for the fact that there are certain appendages which wobble even if you are very thin. It was Sir Robert Helpmann who remarked that the trouble with nude ballet is that there are certain parts of the male anatomy which do not stop when the music does!)

Scientists (who use the word 'obese' to mean fat; I shall use both words in this book) have more complex methods of determining whether or not you are fat (obese) and there is much argument as to the best method.

One method is to weigh the person and compare his weight against his height on a table of standard measurements. The difficulty arises in preparing the table. The most comprehensive set of measurements was drawn up by a group of life insurance companies in America; the heights and weights of over five million life insurance customers were collected, together with the age at which each person died. Tables were then drawn up of so-called desirable weights, which were the weights associated with the longest life span.

There are several criticisms of these tables. They relate to a specific group, namely American people buying life insurance, and this may not represent a typical sample of the population. The figures are now thirty to forty years old and other environmental factors may now operate which did not do so at that time. Some of the measurements were taken in a rather haphazard way, for example heights were measured without the shoes being removed and people were weighed while wearing their clothes. A factor called frame size was introduced without saying exactly how it was defined; indeed it is very difficult to define frame size or to know what contribution it makes to weight. Finally, no allowance was made for age.

In spite of these criticisms, this table still remains the most comprehensive and is the one most frequently used to determine whether a person is obese. For this reason the table is reproduced here. The best way to use it is to take the range for medium frame size for your height and allow yourself 2 or 3 kilograms either side before you decide that you are an undesirable weight! There is a further table, of 'dangerous' weights, on page 19.

The second method used by scientists is the 'skin-fold thickness' method. This is based on the fact that about half of your excess fat is deposited just under the skin. The measurement of skin-fold thickness is widely used in animal husbandry to judge the readiness of animals for market and sophisticated methods are used, such as the passing of an electric current through the skin to determine the electrical resistance of the fat layer and hence its thickness. In humans, a fold of skin is picked up from the underlying muscle and placed for measurement between the two wooden teeth of a skin caliper. There are three sites where skin-fold thickness is commonly measured: the triceps fold on the back of the arm between the shoulder and the elbow; the sub-scapular fold under the winged shoulder bone on the back; and

Table 1 Weights for adults which are associated with longest life span

Men

Height (in shoes)		Small frame		Medium frame		Large frame	
cm	ft in	kg	lb	kg	lb	kg	lb
157·5	5 2	50·8–54·4	112–120	53·5–58·5	118–129	57·2–64	126–141
160	5 3	52·2–55·8	115–123	54·9–60·3	121–133	58·5–65·3	129–144
162·6	5 4	53·5–57·2	118–126	56·2–64·7	124–136	59·9–67·1	132–148
165·1	5 5	54·9–58·5	121–129	57·6–63	127–139	61·2–68·9	135–152
167·6	5 6	56·2–60·3	124–133	59 –64·9	130–143	62·6–70·8	138–156
170·2	5 7	58·1–62·1	128–137	60·8–66·7	134–147	64·4–73	142–161
172·7	5 8	59·9–64	132–141	62·6–68·9	138–152	66·7–75·3	147–166
175·3	5 9	61·7–65·8	136–145	64·4–70·8	142–156	68·5–77·1	151–170
177·8	5 10	63·5–68	140–150	66·2–72·6	146–160	70·3–78·9	155–174
180·3	5 11	65·3–69·9	144–154	68 –74·8	150–165	72·1–81·2	159–179
182·9	6 0	67·1–71·7	148–158	69·9–77·1	154–170	74·4–83·5	164–184
185·4	6 1	68·9–73·5	152–162	71·7–79·4	158–175	76·2–85·7	168–189
188	6 2	70·8–75·7	156–167	73·5–81·6	162–180	78·5–88	173–194
190·5	6 3	72·6–77·6	160–171	75·7–83·5	167–185	80·7–90·3	178–199
193	6 4	74·4–79·4	164–175	78·1–86·2	172–190	82·7–92·5	182–204

Women

Height (in shoes)		Small frame		Medium frame		Large frame	
cm	ft in	kg	lb	kg	lb	kg	lb
147·3	4 10	41·7–44·5	92– 98	43·5–48·5	96–107	47·2–54	104–119
149·9	4 11	42·6–45·8	94–101	44·5–49·9	98–110	48·1–55·3	106–122
152·4	5 0	43·5–47·2	96–104	45·8–51·3	101–113	49·4–56·7	109–125
154·9	5 1	44·9–48·5	99–107	47·2–52·6	104–116	50·8–58·1	112–128
157·5	5 2	46·3–49·9	102–110	48·5–54	107–119	52·2–59·4	115–131
160	5 3	47·6–51·3	105–113	49·9–55·3	110–122	53·5–60·8	118–134
162·6	5 4	49 –52·6	108–116	51·3–57·2	113–126	54·9–62·6	121–138
165·1	5 5	50·3–54	111–119	52·7–59	116–130	56·8–64·4	125–142
167·6	5 6	51·7–55·8	114–123	54·4–61·2	120–135	58·5–66·2	129–146
170·2	5 7	53·5–57·6	118–127	56·2–63	124–139	60·3–68	133–150
172·7	5 8	55·3–59·4	122–131	58·1–64·9	128–143	62·1–69·9	137–154
175·3	5 9	57·2–61·2	126–135	59·9–66·7	132–147	64 –71·7	141–158
177·8	5 10	59 –63·5	130–140	61·7–68·5	136–151	65·8–73·9	145–163
180·3	5 11	60·8–65·3	134–144	63·5–70·3	140–155	67·6–76·2	149–168
182·9	6 0	62·6–67·1	138–148	65·3–72·1	144–159	69·4–78·5	153–173

Source: modified from Metropolitan Life Insurance Company, Statistical Bulletin, 41 (1960).

the abdominal fold on the abdomen. The skin caliper tends to give inconsistent results, depending on the skill and experience of the user. However, it has been used with some success in large community surveys to identify malnourished children in countries in the Third World when there is an imminent threat of famine.

More accurate ways to measure obesity are methods which measure fat, and only fat. Weight measurements in trained athletes, for example, will give the wrong answers about obesity because the highly developed muscle will be included in the weight. One way to measure the actual fat content of the body is to use Archimedes' principle and determine the density by weighing the body first in air and then totally submerged in water. For large populations the method is too cumbersome. On a personal level, anyone attending an obesity clinic is likely to regard the suggestion of total submersion as signifying rather misplaced evangelical zeal.

To sum up, most methods only tell you where you fit within the population at the present time. Populations change. Clothing manufacturers find that their most popular selling size is larger now than it was twenty years ago. To those who wonder if they are fat, I would say this. It's like love: if you *feel* fat, you *are* fat; if you are not sure, then it's probably not the real thing!

How does it happen?

Let's take my mother's ideas first. Her first theory, when she saw a thin person eating a mountain of food, was 'he must have worms'. Even in an affluent community there are worms, and many children will wake up one night scratching their bottom, a sign that they have roundworm infestation. (The worms come out at night to lay their eggs.) But the nutritional status of these children is good, and they are not underweight despite quite heavy infestation. In other communities where food is sparse, and the children have a heavy infestation of worms in their gut, the children are very thin. However, the reason is that their food is deficient in energy, protein, or vitamins. Worms alone do not make you thin.

My mother's second theory was that it was all in the glands. Our neighbour's boy was obese, a roly-poly child shunned by the other children; his mother gave him lots of sweets to make up for the fact that he had no one to play with. He would sit on the gate, muching his way through his umpteenth chocolate bar. He went into the army when he was a teenager, away from his mother's sweets, and doing hard physical work. He emerged a slim svelte figure. 'They must have taken his glands out', said my mother.

It is true that a malfunction in any one of the endocrine glands may produce a change in weight. For example, under-production of thyroid hormone leads to overweight, along with a sluggishness and a hypersensitivity to cold. An excess of the steroid hormones also leads to obesity of a special kind, with fat deposited mainly on the trunk and a puffiness in the face; patients 'on steroids' often look fat. In none of these cases, however, is obesity the major feature. In 1980 studies on grossly obese women (more than twice ideal weight) suggested that their obesity may be attributable to an abnormal response of one of the pituitary hormones. Such a condition is very rare: in 999 cases out of 1,000 you cannot blame obesity on your glands.

Lastly, my mother would say that the thin people are 'poor-doers'. On the farm, these are animals which fail to thrive in spite of eating well; their opposites are the animals which become plump and glossy and ready for market in the twinkling of an eye, the 'good-doers'. The argument is that in the good-doers all the food is absorbed and used, but in the poor-doers most of it passes through the intestine and out in the faeces and is wasted.

There is no evidence that this happens in man. In normal healthy man, everything that is eaten is absorbed, the only exception being uncooked vegetables, where the cell walls are incompletely broken down. There are malabsorption diseases, in which there is a defect of the intestinal walls which results in some of the food passing through the intestine without being absorbed. These diseases are rare, and the difference between the good-doers and the poor-doers has to be explained in some other way. (One of my mother's best friends had one of these diseases, called tropical sprue. She was given a special allowance of bananas during the war and I remember seeing a large bowl of this practically unknown fruit on her table. My mother's diagnosis for her friend's thinness was not that she was a poor-doer, but that she worried too much!)

Having dealt with the fallacies, what about the facts? How

do you get fat? There is no mystery about this. A fat person is fat because at some stage he has been in positive energy balance: that is, he has eaten more food than was needed to cover his energy expenditure, and he has stored the excess as fat. Having done this, if he then reduces his food intake to match his current energy expenditure, he will not get any fatter, but the fat he has gained will remain. To get rid of it, he must go into negative energy balance; that is, he must eat less food than he needs, and then his metabolism will use the stored fat in his body, and he will lose weight.

This explains why fat people often appear to eat and exercise to the same extent as thin people: in each case, a status quo is being maintained. To shift the status quo, that is to lose weight, you have to starve yourself (see next chapter).

The real question is: why do some people stay thin with no effort, while for others it is a constant battle? The answer to this question is not known at present, although it may be discovered in the future. We may find that there are very small differences in metabolism that explain it, such as the recent demonstration of differences between fat and thin people in the way they adapt to cold temperatures, differences which are related to metabolic differences in the brown fat in their bodies. Another suggestion is that everyone has a sort of 'heavistat' which sets his appetite at a level which results in a set weight for that individual. There may be important psychological reasons for overweight, for example, many people tend to eat more when they are unhappy and distressed: they seem to eat for comfort, and this behaviour may have been produced by having received food as a reward when they were young. Heredity may play a role, although it is difficult to separate heredity from environment as a cause: it has often been pointed out that although fat parents often have fat children, they also tend to have fat adopted children and fat pets.

Whatever the reasons, the difference does exist. If you are one of the naturally fat ones, it will be of small comfort to you to know that the scientists cannot tell you why. At the present time, however, there is no single theory which satisfactorily explains this well-recognized difference between those who find it easy and those who don't!

Is it wrong to be fat?

It takes courage today to be like Ma Larkins: fat, and happy to be fat. Everywhere there is pressure to be thin; fashion models are thin, cinema stars are thin, the figures that look at us from the television screen are thin. Enormous effort is spent on getting thin, people follow diets and they join slimming clubs. If money is no object, there are health farms where it costs a fortune to enjoy a discipline, exercise regime, and diet not unlike those offered in prison. Why? Is there a need for this obsession? What are the advantages of being thin, or the disadvantages of being fat?

When people ask the question 'Is it wrong to be fat?' they are usually asking one of two things: either 'Will I die sooner if I am fat?' or 'Am I so fat that you might stop loving me?'

Let's take the health question first. In order to answer this, you have to take a very large number of people, weigh them all, put them into fat or non-fat groups; then wait for them to die and see whether the fat ones die earlier than the thin ones. Apart from the difficulty in measuring fatness, which I have already described, there are many other problems associated with such a study, not the least of these being the time span involved. Some subjects included will not die for many years after the project is begun. That means that since the investigator who begins such a study often has no results for many years, there are no quick returns such as scientific honours, promotion, grant money, or conference trips. Consequently, studies like this tend to be left to public bodies or financially interested companies. The two most complete studies are the Framingham Study and the Metropolitan Life Insurance Study.

The first of these was carried out in Framingham, Massachusetts, sponsored by the government of the United States of America. The study involved about 6,000 men and women selected at random from the normal population of the town. Each person was examined medically twice a year and a general record of his health was kept (including weight). Signs and symptoms of cardio-vascular disease were especially noted. The study commenced in 1949 and is still in progress. Results have led to the conclusion that people who suffer from obesity had a greater chance of getting angina (heart pain) or suffering from sudden death from a heart attack. However, the body weight has to be *20 per cent above average* before such risks become apparent. If high blood pressure or raised cholesterol levels are also present, the risk of dying is greatly increased.

The second study was a retrospective one carried out by the Metropolitan Life Insurance Company in America. Over 100,000 customers who had bought life insurance policies were followed up thirty years later to see whether those who were obese at the time of buying the policy had died at a younger age than those who were not obese. It was found that the obese subjects did die younger, but that the effect was not significant unless the body weight exceeded the desirable figure by more than 30 per cent.

People who exceeded these limits were found to be susceptible to several diseases. Firstly, there was a greater chance of developing diabetes of the milder form, which develops in middle age and can often be controlled by diet or drugs administered by mouth, without the need of insulin injections. Secondly, obese people run a greater risk of developing gallstones. (The well-known student crib of the five 'f's' characteristic of the gallbladder patient takes this into account: fair, female, forty, fertile, and FAT.) Thirdly, the very obese patient will often have difficulty in breathing and may become very drowsy because he underbreathes. Such a patient is described in the *Pickwick Papers* ('Goodness me, is that boy asleep again!'); the description is so accurate that the disease has been named the Pickwickian syndrome. The difficulty in breathing also means that there is an increased risk if the patient has to have an anaesthetic. Lastly, fat people suffer more from heart disease.

However, the Life Insurance Study confirmed the results of the Framingham Study: obesity alone, unless it is gross, does not seem to be a factor which increases the risk of heart disease; but if other factors predisposing to heart disease are present (family history, smoking, lack of exercise, high blood cholesterol, high blood pressure: see Ch. 16) then obesity increases the risk.

Since these studies, two other complications of obesity have been recognized. One is the greatly increased risk of osteoarthritis. The stress placed by the extra weight on the joints, particularly the hip and the knee, produces degenerative changes which cause the joint to break down. The other risk is that obese people have a greater incidence of kidney stones than non-obese people.

In trying to sum up the situation, I think the fairest thing to say is this: if you are mildly obese, that is not more than 20 per cent overweight, you run a negligible risk. This means, in very rough figures, that your weight for your height should never exceed that given in the following table of *maximum* safe weights. If your weight DOES exceed the value given (and note, these are

Table 2 Maximum weights compatible with normal life expectancy

Women

Height			Weight	
cm	ft	in	kg	lb
145	4	9	53	117
147	4	10	55	121
150	4	11	57	125
152	5	0	59	129
155	5	1	60	132
157	5	2	61	135
160	5	3	63	139
163	5	4	65	143
165	5	5	67	148
168	5	6	69	152
170	5	7	71	157
173	5	8	74	162
175	5	9	76	167
178	5	10	78	172
180	5	11	80	177

Men

Height			Weight	
cm	ft	in	kg	lb
157	5	2	68	914
160	5	3	69	152
163	5	4	71	156
165	5	5	72	159
168	5	6	74	163
170	5	7	76	168
173	5	8	79	173
175	5	9	81	178
178	5	10	83	183
180	5	11	85	188
183	6	0	88	194
185	6	1	90	199
188	6	2	92	203
190	6	3	95	210
193	6	4	99	217

not ideal weights, they are the *upper limit* of safe weights) you stand a statistically higher chance of dying earlier than your thinner brothers. In addition, you increase your chances of having diabetes, gall-stones, breathing difficulties, heart disease, osteo-arthritis, and kidney stones.

Now let's turn to the other question: 'Am I so fat that you might stop loving me?' In the twentieth century, television and magazine advertisements reinforce the view that it is desirable to be slim. This is not so in all communities. In a certain tribe in Africa, the women are not considered marriageable unless they are enormously fat, and puny would-be brides are put into cages to be fattened up so that they might invite a prospective spouse's loving glances. Nor has it always been true in our own culture. A fashionable and beautiful young lady painted by Rubens would weigh twice as much as a fashionable and beautiful young lady photographed by *Vogue* magazine today, yet each represents the contemporary ideal. Fashion dictates the answer to the question. In Western cultures today, if you are fat, people will tend to stop loving you.

There are experiments which demonstrate this attitude. A group of children was asked to rate a series of six pictures of other children in order of attractiveness. The pictures showed children who were similar except that each had a different physical disability; the first had a left hand missing, the second a disfigured mouth, the third had crutches and a brace on his leg, the fourth was a in a wheelchair, the fifth was fat. The sixth picture showed a normal child. The pictures were placed in front of a child who was asked to select the one he would like best as his friend, then that picture was removed and the child was asked again until all the pictures had been chosen. Overwhelmingly, the fat child was liked the least. When the study was repeated with adults, the results were exactly the same. Studies of this kind are often difficult to interpret for all sorts of reasons, but the low rating of the obese child was so universal in this study that it is very hard to avoid the conclusion that fat people are not loved and that there is a social stigma against them.

Before I leave this subject, I would like to return to the original question 'Is it wrong to be fat?' I used the word 'wrong' with its connotation of morality because it seems to me that the whole question of obesity has become tinged with puritanic over-tones. Mild obesity, say up to 20 per cent overweight, which is the type suffered by most people who are on the slimming treadmill, is not seriously detrimental to health. It is, however, a social dis-advantage and the idea that it is *wrong* to be fat is supported wholeheartedly by the diet-food industry, the profit-making slimming clubs, and anyone else who stands to gain financially from making people feel bad about being fat. This produces a river of money which never dries up, because obesity is, in all but a few exceptional cases, an incurable disease.

There is nothing 'wrong' with being slightly obese, it simply means that you do not conform to the values demanded by a relatively media-dominated society. However, obesity beyond the magic 20 per cent is detrimental to health, and should be cor-rected or avoided. Its correction or avoidance are the subjects of the following chapter.

3 How to lose weight

If you decide that you want to lose weight either for aesthetic or for health reasons, how do you do it? There are only two ways, and they are both related to the energy balance discussed in Chapter 1. You must either eat less or exercise more: how to do so is the subject of this chapter. Firstly, however, there are three popular fallacies about losing weight.

Fallacies

Massage has long been practised in the belief that it reduces weight. If you are a 'do-it-yourself' enthusiast you can even buy a little electric vibrator which you run over the appropriate areas. Otherwise you employ a masseur and it is the masseur who will lose the weight, as the work requires a great deal of physical energy. For the client, there will be no magical melting away of fat, no redistribution of weight, and no sudden toning up of muscle. There may possibly be certain fringe benefits, and while these may be highly pleasurable in themselves, they will do nothing to lessen the problem of obesity.

Turkish baths feature in gangster films as a particularly unpleasant way of doing away with the villain; you locked the door and turned up the heat, leaving him to die most uncomfortably. They, and their close cousin the sauna, also enjoy a less evil role as a means of reducing weight. They unquestionably do produce weight loss; the scales at your feet as you step out of the hot room bear witness to that. However, the weight loss is made up entirely of sweat, which consists of water and certain salts and no fat at all. The lost fluid leads to thirst and is replaced as soon as possible, which explains why commercial establishments always weigh you straight after the Turkish bath and before you reach the bar. This method of weight reduction is of short-term use; for example, for those sportsmen who have to weigh in, such as jockeys or boxers. In the long term it is useless. Equally useless are the small plastic garments which are worn around the waist, upper arm, or thigh, and which are supposed to melt away the fat in specific places.

Drugs of various kinds have been used to promote slimming. At one time, capsules were sold which contained the eggs of intestinal worms, these hatched out in the intestine and were supposed to eat the food you ate and thus prevent you from getting fat. (No one ever explained why a lot of fat worms in your intestines did not make you fat.) On a less macabre but more dangerous note, thyroid tablets were sold with the idea of increasing metabolic rate and so leading to weight loss. At worst they were potentially dangerous, at best they were useless, as the body simply decreased its own production of thyroid hormone to compensate.

The drugs used at present are the anorexigenic drugs, which are claimed to suppress appetitite. Many of the ones presently available are addictive, being related to the 'pep pill', Dexedrine. For this reason they are dangerous and should be used only if the excess weight endangers the health of the patient, and then only under strict medical supervision. Other drugs used (for example, Ponderax, Mazindol) are not addictive but may have other unwanted side-effects such as producing sleepiness. In view of these side-effects and of the difficulty of proving the effectiveness of such drugs on appetite control, it would seem wise to limit their use.

Eat less food

Reduction of intake of food is one of the two procedures which *do* reduce body weight (the other is increase in physical activity, which will be discussed next). Until quite recently, overeating was thought to be the commonest cause of overweight. The fat man would cry plaintively 'but I don't eat as much as you do', thereby condemning himself in the eyes of his thin friend as a liar as well as a glutton. Careful observation has now vindicated his claim by establishing that, on the whole, fat people do eat less than thin people. However, in any weight-reduction programme eating less should play a role, and this is how to go about it.

Firstly, you should realize that it is not easy. This fact is known to everyone who has ever tried to diet, but it is rarely admitted or even hinted at in the glossy advertisements of slimming foods and diets. In order to lose weight, you have to eat less food than that required to provide the energy you need, so that the body is forced to use its own larder of fat. This means that any weight-reduction programme relying on reduced food intake will produce a state of discomfort, which will vary from mild to acute depending on how much you love your food. If you are prepared to face this fact read on, if not, learn to live with your plumpness.

Secondly, there is no such thing as a slimming food. That is, nothing that you eat, including grapefruit juice, will melt the fat away. At best, the material you eat will contain no available energy (methyl cellulose and water come into this category) or very little energy (green vegetables, for example, but even they will make you fat if you eat enough of them). So don't fall for the advertising of preparations reputed to be slimming: the only thing that will get slim is your purse!

Thirdly, special diets are often inadequate, frequently expensive, and always impossible to maintain. I remember one woman saying nervously to me: 'I do hope my husband doesn't go on a diet again; we can't afford it.' His diet consisted of fillet steak, chicken breasts, and prawns, with a little caviar if the palate became jaded. Another time, on enquiring why a friend looked so harassed, I learned that he could not remember whether today was the first egg day or the second chicken day: any weight loss he sustained was due to the worry of remembering which stage he had reached! Life is too short to think carefully every time you put something into your mouth and anyway, who wants to give up steak and kidney pudding for boiled chicken?

The best long-term attack is to stick to your normal diet and to eat less of it. This assumes that your normal diet is reasonably varied; in any case, it could hardly contain less essential nutrients than some of the diets which are 'guaranteed' to help you lose weight. All day and every day, eat two-thirds the quantity that you would normally eat. Every time you sit down to a meal, think of the amount you would usually eat and take two-thirds of that amount. Eat anything you want to, but eat less of it. Adopt this habit of eating less and gradually your habits will change, and eating less will become a pattern that will persist. It will never be easy, but it will stand a higher chance of success than a special diet.

In case this sounds like a lifetime of misery, remember that once your weight is down to the level you are aiming at, you can increase your food intake to a less Spartan level. During the weight-losing period, part of your energy must come from your own body fat. Once you have used up enough of your own fat, this energy can come from food and you can therefore eat slightly more.

If you are the sort of person who likes communal activity, responds to authority, and has a little money to spare, join a slimming group, such as Weightwatchers International, Silhouette, or a similar organization. I don't agree with everything they say (nor would they agree with everything I say) but they have a sensible, realistic approach to dieting and they can be very helpful to those of us who find it difficult to sustain the effort on our own.

Lastly, here are a few hints to help.

1. Be honest. It's no good cutting down to two-thirds if you have multiplied by 2 first!
2. Remember, all alcoholic drinks have energy and are potentially fattening.
3. Never let yourself get really hungry. Eat little and often, never miss breakfast, snack between meals if you want to, but have smaller snacks.
4. Learn which are the really energy-dense foods, so that you can avoid them unless you really love them. All the fats, including *chocolate*, are in this category.
5. Learn which low-energy foods you enjoy, so that you can 'binge' if you feel like it. Such things as tomatoes and apples; clear soup; *small* gin diluted with lots of low-Calorie tonic or ditto whisky and soda; cottage cheese (when compared with all other cheeses); all the cabbage family; boiled sweets if you are a sweet tooth because they can be sucked and therefore last longer; jam for diabetics if you love jam; yogurt instead of cream.

6. Don't be fooled by claims of weight losses of 3 to 4 kilograms (6 to 8 lb) per week.* Five hundred grams (1 lb) per week is the realistic level to aim for, producing a negative energy balance of about 2,700 kJ (650 kcal) per day. This can be achieved by reducing your present food intake by a quarter, *or* a daily walk of about 10 kilometres (6 m.), or some combination of both.

Do more exercise

In the previous chapter I described differences between 'active' and 'inactive' people. If you suspect that you belong to the inactive group, what can you do about it? You almost certainly cannot change your personality; such behavioural patterns are probably established irrevocably by adulthood. Your aim must be consciously to introduce some physical activity into your life.

The maximum energy a fit man or woman can spend at a stretch is in the region of 1,250 kJ (300 kcal). The following activities would spend that much:

> Half an hour of fast squash
> An hour of continuous swimming
> Walking 6 kilometres (4 miles) briskly
> Jogging for forty-five minutes
> A two-hour round of golf

One of these activities performed *each day* would result in a weekly weight loss of 200 grams (7 oz.). Such a level of activity is, however, beyond most of us: we would be happy to accomplish it once or twice a week! Even then it takes a great deal of will-power: your partner drops out; your spouse arranges a social engagement; it's too cold in winter; there are all sorts of excuses and you gradually give it up.

---

* For those interested in the figures, a weight loss of 4 kilograms (8 lb) in one week represents a negative energy balance of 150,000 kJ (36,000 kcal). To achieve this, you would have to spend a whole week *eating nothing, and indulging in strenuous physical activity for six hours a day*. So what about the people who claim to have done it? The explanation is that on a very low-carbohydrate diet, the body uses up the stored carbohydrate (muscle glycogen). Stored with this carbohydrate is a lot of water, 4 to 6 grams of water for every gram of carbohydrate. A loss of 4 kilograms includes 3 kilograms of water, and as soon as any carbohydrate is eaten, this water is regained. This explains the initial rapid weight loss on any low-carbohydrate diet.

Far more effective, from the point of view of losing weight, is to find a way of building exercise into your everyday life. I give here a list of suggestions. Select those which best suit your lifestyle, and possibly these will suggest others to you.

1. *Find some way of walking.* Of all the advice to the would-be-slim, I think this is the most important. Could you walk to work? Or even part way? Go out at lunchtime and explore your neighbourhood. Aim at 3 kilometres (2 m.) per day; over a year that is equivalent to losing about 7 kilograms (15 lb) of body fat.

2. Never use a lift or an elevator. Even if you are going to the tenth floor, try the stairs.

3. Take up vegetable gardening. You will improve your diet as well as your figure.

4. If you are paying someone to do any physical task for you, stop! Wash your own car, do some of your own housework, mow your own lawns. Next time your motor mower breaks down, don't kick it, buy an old-fashioned mechanical one that you have to push.

5. Choose a holiday that is active – walking, skiing if you can afford it, swimming if it is warm enough.

6. Buy a dog, a big one that needs lots of exercise (and which will discourage unwanted attentions from strangers if your only chance of walking is in a city at night-time).

7. If you have children, invent one 'activity thing' to do with them at week-ends. Challenge them at tennis, roller skating, swimming, or even running. If you choose something that is fun, the children will keep you up to it. (If you have no children, borrow some; their parents will love a rest!)

8. Don't say that you are too busy. Go to bed half an hour later or get up half an hour earlier. Use the time to do something active: if you used it for walking, even round the house, that would be 7 kilograms (15 lb) per year.

4 Starvation

Starvation occurs when an individual is eating food with an energy value insufficient to supply his needs. He is in negative energy balance.

There are many degrees of starvation, with effects ranging from a small check in the growth rate of children to the terrible wasting disease seen in famine. It is often said that half the world has too little to eat and the other half too much. The United Nations has estimated the number of underfed people at 400 millions, but complete surveys have never been carried out and no one knows exactly how many people in the world have too little food. What we do know is that there are millions of such people and that little effective help can be, or is being, given to them.

This chapter describes some of the features of starvation; its causes, its effects, and its treatment. The increasing size of the problem demands a more rational approach to its solution and this in turn means re-education of the people in rich countries; this crucial problem is discussed in the section on the prevention of famine. Finally, there are two bizarre forms of starvation which are seen even in rich countries – fasting for political reasons and anorexia nervosa – in which the patients show the same effects as those seen in famine; these two situations are described at the end of the chapter.

Famine

Famine is a constant threat in some areas of the world where population growth has outstripped food production. The situation will continue until food production is increased, or population growth is controlled. In the threatened areas, shortage of food is always present and is precipitated into famine by various events. These events have occurred regularly in the past and they are easily identified. They are: drought, crop pests, natural disasters such as flood or earthquake, and war. (The last cause is as old as the rest; only its methods change. In biblical times, starvation was produced by siege; in the eighteenth century the scorched-earth policy of the Napoleonic Wars decimated the Russian peasantry by producing famine; and the defoliation policies used in our own time have had a similar effect.)

In such cases the effects of starvation are tragically obvious. Undernutrition on a smaller scale is not so easy to identify, and yet it is important to identify it so that steps may be taken to prevent its effects. Many sophisticated procedures have been tried to test whether a child is malnourished, such as the analysis of blood and urine; but none of these has proved satisfactory in the field. The simple tests which involve measuring the children seem to work best. The 'height-for-age' and the 'weight-for-height' are two such tests, in which the child's height and weight are compared with those of normal children of the same age. When your schoolchild says 'the nurse came to school and measured me' it means that the nutritional state of children is being monitored even in our affluent community. In poor communities such vigilance is even more important. The only apparatus needed is a set of scales, a measuring rule, and charts giving values for normal children. These tests are used by the World Health Organisation field teams to detect undernourished children in poor countries.

The effects of starvation

Classically, there are two diseases of starvation. The first is marasmus, in which the patient is simply not getting enough to eat. He is in negative energy balance. The second is kwashiorkor, in which there is enough to eat, but there is a deficiency of protein. Kwashiorkor was described in 1932 by Cicely Williams, the first woman medical officer appointed in East Africa. It occurred usually when a child was no longer breast-fed and was weaned on to adult food (the name means literally the 'sickness the older child gets when the next baby is born').

It is being increasingly recognized that the distinction between marasmus and kwashiorkor is not always clear cut.

Kwashiorkor is not a common disease and may be limited to areas where the staple diet is the low-protein root, cassava. When an undersized child is found in a famine situation, there are no definite tests to show whether the main deficiency is protein or energy; usually, both are deficient. For these reasons, terms coming into more general use are Protein-Calorie-Malnutrition (PCM), or Protein-Energy-Malnutrition (PEM).

In communities where PEM is widespread, the situation is often complicated by other factors such as lack of vitamins, presence of infectious diseases, and the presence of worms and other parasites in the gut. For these reasons, it is impossible to give a simple picture of the symptoms. However, there are certain striking features always present, some affecting the body, and others which may affect the brain.

In the body, the most obvious change is loss of weight. The fat disappears and the muscles waste away; the skin becomes too big for the body and falls into folds and wrinkles; the eyes seem large because they occupy a larger space proportionally as the fat and muscle around them disappear; the bones protrude so that previously hidden structures like the hip joint, the ribs, and the elbow joint become clearly visible. Less apparent, but potentially more dangerous, is the loss of tissue in internal organs such as the gut and the heart. The heart may shrink to one-third of its normal size, leaving insufficient heart muscle to pump blood around the body. The gut can lose so much tissue that it becomes quite transparent; during post-mortems carried out on victims of starvation the contents of the gut are often visible through the paper-like walls. The effect of this loss of tissue is to reduce the capacity of the gut to digest and absorb food, so that when food does become available it passes straight through. The changes in both of these organs may contribute to the death of the patient even after treatment has been started; many starvation victims die in hospital from heart failure.

This loss of weight is due to the fact that the body is literally using its own tissue for energy. Fat is the largest source. The metabolism of fat, if there is no carbohydrate to metabolize with it, produces acid substances which may produce coma and death. These substances give the breath and urine a characteristic smell (in some low-carbohydrate slimming diets they are tested for in the urine by using strips of special indicator paper). Body protein is also burnt for energy, and this produces the depletion of vital organs like the heart and the gut.

Superimposed on these physical changes are possible changes to the intellect of the growing child. This is suggested by observations that children of famine appear dull and listless and may be retarded intellectually. Experiments on animals suggest that there are critical periods of brain growth during development, and that if food is restricted during these critical periods, the brain might not develop normally.

Other experiments, however, suggest that famine does not permanently affect intellect. For example, examination of the brain from victims of starvation shows that it is spared during starvation when compared with other organs, showing negligible weight loss. In another investigation, intelligence was measured in adults who had been born during the German occupation of Holland during the Second World War. These individuals had been born to mothers who were starving, and had suffered severe starvation themselves over the first few months or years of their lives, yet as adults they showed no intellectual impairment when compared with a normal population. These results suggest that even if mental retardation does occur in famine, children can 'catch up' on their mental growth when the famine is over.

The question of the effect of famine on intellect is therefore unresolved, because famine is a complex situation and food supply may not be the only problem. For example, in a famine mothers may be too listless and apathetic to spend time playing with their children. This may contribute to the slow mental development of the child; it is possible that the dull intellect of the children of famine is due to lack of stimulation in their immediate environment, and that it can be corrected when the famine ends. However, in the absence of specific proof to the contrary, it is necessary to suspect that famine not only may affect its immediate victims, but that it may also produce a future generation with impaired intellect.

Treatment

The short-term treatment of starvation seems obvious: give food. The situation is not so simple.

Ordinary food can be damaging, as was seen, for example, after the war in concentration camps, when many starving prisoners suffered severe diarrhoea and gastro-intestinal upsets because they were given whatever food was available, and this sometimes meant bully beef and baked beans! In wealthy communities, isolated cases of starvation can be treated initially by intravenous feeding, with careful monitoring of salt and sugar levels in the blood. This is continued until the salt balance has been corrected and the patient is a little stronger. A simple diet of bland food, usually in a liquid form, may then be started, and gradually the diet is changed to normal food. In situations where thousands are starving, intravenous feeding is not possible. A simple, cheap mixture has to be found which is easily digested and palatable. In the African famines, relief workers have successfully used a mixture of dried skim milk, corn oil, and sugar, emulsified into a thick mixture like a milk shake.

One might imagine that once food is available, the problem is over, but many people who are treated still die. As already described, the gut is so thin and wasted that food may not be absorbed; the heart is too small and the patient gets heart failure; diarrhoea develops and will not respond to treatment; organs like the liver and the kidney and the pancreas are smaller; and all normal metabolic processes are threatened. Sometimes victims of starvation may survive for months with good nursing care, and then die.

Sound nutritional principles have not always been observed in international efforts to treat famine. For example, for many years it was the practice to rush high-protein food (often skimmed milk from rich countries with a dairy surplus) into famine areas in the belief that protein deficiency was the main problem. Then the dairy surplus dried up, and enormous sums of money were spent (and made!) developing high-protein foods. However, as I pointed out previously, the prime function of food is to provide energy, and a starving man will utilize protein for energy, not for body-building; these programmes therefore represent an expensive way of providing energy. In order to spread the limited resources further, recent policy has been to supply grain. This is much more economical than providing high-protein food. It fills the main requirement (for energy) and provides some protein as well. The food provided has to be similar to the familiar staple food of the community; if it is not, local or religious custom may prevent its consumption. There are many reports of rice-eating people dying of starvation while the granaries were full of wheat.

In addition, there are enormous administrative problems peculiar to famine situations. Communications break down and transport of large quantities of food is very difficult. Local black markets develop and food is withheld from those who need it by members of their own community. The situation is complicated by terrible decisions; often the worst affected victims are beyond help and must be left to die while the limited resources are used to help those less badly affected. Treatment often involves moving a child into hospital, where he may die from infections picked up in the hospital environment, such as measles. Once treated, he has to be returned to his home and the starvation problem reappears.

If I have made the situation look hopeless, it is because present attempts have failed to solve the problem of short-term aid. The granaries of America and the food stores of Europe are full of surplus food. The Third World is full of starving people. So far, efforts to bring one to the other have been, at best, only partially successful. Hope lies in the self-help schemes, where dedicated helpers are prepared to go into the community, find local solutions to local problems, and teach the community how to apply them. Two examples illustrate this. In East Africa, a missionary started his own vegetable garden, and taught the villagers how to start theirs: when famine came, these villagers survived because they had vegetables to supplement the meagre supply of grain. In India, a well had dried up and a new deeper one was built with help from a locally based World Health Organisation team; water from the new well provided irrigation and made the community much less dependent on the arrival of rain. Schemes such as these cost very little, they give permanent help, they save lives, and, most important of all, they allow people to come to terms with their own environment and survive within it.

Prevention of famine

The problem of providing effective aid to a community in a

famine, coupled with the obvious anomaly of having half the world starving while the other half overeats, has led many people to ask whether something cannot be done to correct the situation. Recent thoughts on this question challenge long-held beliefs in the inherent superiority of Western diets and agricultural policies.

Platitudes mouthed by the politicians are often not true, but they tend to become accepted as truths. America as the bread-basket of the Third World, for example: yet most of America's surplus grain goes to other highly developed countries like Russia and Europe. The greater efficiency of Western farming methods is another example: yet in the highly developed countries it takes 5 to 10 kilojoules of energy to produce each kilojoule in the food harvested; whereas in the so-called primitive societies, only one-fifth of a kilojoule is spent for every kilojoule harvested. Has this 'development' taken us along the wrong path?

In a book called *The Famine Business* Colin Tudge sums up these thoughts in a provocative and highly readable argument. Read the book if you have the opportunity. Many of the ideas in the following paragraphs are taken from it.

One of the main features of diet in developed countries is the increase in the consumption of animal protein. Since animal protein is nearly always associated with a high proportion of animal fat (and indeed, fat animals are favoured by the breeder), this is bad for our health. In addition, it is very wasteful since the animal has to be fed on plant protein to make its own protein, and it does the conversion very inefficiently. Tudge quotes the example of the Americans who give their livestock around 20 million tonnes of protein a year in a form that could perfectly well be eaten by human beings (this means grain). The livestock in turn produce about 2 million tonnes of protein. The 18 million tonne loss is equivalent to 90 per cent of the yearly world protein deficit.

A more rational use of the land would be to grow protein in the form of cereals and beans (pulses), and to graze animals only on those areas which are unsuitable for cultivation. In addition, grazing beasts should be bred for lean size rather than fat size. Alcohol, for which there is no nutritional necessity, and vege-tables, should be produced to add variety to our diets and pleasure to our lives. In the crucial chapter in his book (the chapter called 'Rational Agriculture'), Tudge argues this case.

Are such ideas nutritionally sound? Indeed they are. Potatoes and grain are both good sources of protein; the protein to carbohydrate ratio is about 1 to 5, which is right for human needs. Pulses contain those amino acids which wheat lacks and are therefore a perfect complement to bread. (This idea of complementary proteins is discussed in Chapter 7 on proteins.) Pulses and grain have no animal fat; and a high fibre content if they are not processed first; two nutritional advantages. So we would all be healthier if we ate such a diet. In addition, used in this way, the land resources of the world would be sufficient to feed its increasing population. Each country could become more self-supporting: Britain, for example, can produce enough grain to support its people but needs to import grain at present since so much is fed to its livestock.

Such ideas will not be readily accepted. Moving from a 'peasant' to a 'sophisticated' diet is a sign to many of us that we have succeeded in life; a move back to beans and mash would seem like an admission of failure. A greater knowledge in the community of the facts of nutrition and an increasing awareness of the dangers of the typical diet in affluent countries may change this view. Otherwise it looks seriously as though we might all starve to death.

Fasting

Professional fasting men have acted as curiosities for a ghoulish public for many years. Ghandi made famous the use of fasting for political ends when he went without food to protest against the British rule in India. The Suffragettes were another group who fasted for political reasons, refusing food when they were imprisoned. This led to the practice of force-feeding, in which the woman was held while a tube was pushed into her throat and food was poured in. It took several people to restrain the unwilling victim; the process was degrading both to the victim and to those carrying it out. Apart from this, there were dangers associated with the possible passage of the food into the lungs due to the lodging of the tube in the windpipe instead of the oesophagus. The process has been discontinued in many countries – in Britain, for example, prisoners who fast are counselled and, if they are adamant, they are allowed to die.

How long does it take to die? In a healthy, non-obese man, given free access to water but no food at all, and undertaking no physical activity, death occurs after about fifty days. He requires energy during this time to carry out his basal metabolic processes; this takes about 6,000 kJ (1,500 kcal) per day. This energy is obtained from his own body stores. A negligible amount comes from stored carbohydrate. Most comes from body fat, and the remainder comes from protein as he metabolizes his own muscle tissue for energy. When his body weight is down to three-quarters of its normal level, he still has every chance of recovery. But once he drops to half his normal weight recovery is less likely, even with the most careful medical treatment. During the latter days of his fast he will feel unwell and lethargic. Eventually he will pass into a coma, and then he will die.

Anorexia nervosa

This type of voluntary fasting usually occurs in young women, often after a slimming diet. The subject may refuse all food, or may vomit immediately after food is eaten so that none of it is absorbed. Sometimes very large doses of purgatives are taken and the bowel becomes so active that the food passes through without being absorbed. The weight falls to extremely low levels, menstruation ceases, and, if untreated, the patient may literally starve herself to death. The basis of the disease is a psychological disorder, and the reasons for it developing are very complex and probably different in every case. Its cure depends on careful and skilled treatment and counselling. It is almost certainly outside the power of the family to initiate help: expert advice must be sought (although the family may play a very important role once treatment is commenced). If you know anyone who has this disorder, you should arrange for him or her to see a doctor.

5 Carbohydrates

During the last century we have discovered that the food we eat is made up of carbohydrates, fats, and proteins, together with vitamins and minerals. The chemical structure of each of these is known. The chemical composition is known even for various flavours: the flavour of bacon, for example, can be imitated in the test tube, so that we can manufacture crisps that taste like bacon, biscuits that taste like bacon, and snacks that taste like bacon; the only thing we seem to have trouble with is bacon that tastes like bacon!

Carbohydrates, fats, proteins, vitamins, and minerals: each one plays its role in metabolism, each is necessary to maintain health. In the following chapters, the particular function of each one is described, together with its harmful effects (if any) and the foods which contain it.

What is carbohydrate?

Carbohydrates are manufactured by plants, which are able to use solar energy, air, and water, and trap this energy in food. Animals are unable to do this, which means that ultimately every one of us is dependent on plants for our existence.

The carbohydrate manufactured by the plant exists in three different forms. The first product made is a simple sugar. However, large quantities of sugar are not found in plants, except in sugar cane and sugar beet; the plant normally turns the sugar into starch, the second kind of carbohydrate. Or it may convert it into fibres and supporting structures, such as cellulose, which make up the third group.

The simplest type of carbohydrate is therefore a sugar. Glucose is a sugar; others are fructose, the sugar found in fruit; lactose, which is milk sugar; honey, which is various sugars in solution; and manna, the sap of the tamarisk tree which sustained the Israelites when they crossed the dessert in biblical times. By far the commonest sugar, however, is sucrose, or ordinary domestic sugar, which comes from sugar cane or sugar beet. All sugars have two characteristics which distinguish them from the other two types of carbohydrate: firstly, they taste sweet, which makes many people want to eat more of them, and secondly, there is accumulating evidence that too much of them may harm you (see page 40).

The second type of carbohydrate is called a polysaccharide (literally, many sugars) and consists of a combination of thousands of sugar molecules. The commonest example is starch. The great advantage to plants of making polysaccharides is that the molecules are too big to leak out through the holes in the cell membrane (unlike sugar molecules), so that once a starch molecule is formed, it stays inside the cell. This makes the starches an ideal form in which to store energy for future use; for example, food stored in this way in the seed enables the plant to start growing again in the spring. This characteristic of the plant is used by man to his advantage when he harvests the plant in the autumn for his own food. Considerable skill and energy have been expended by botanists to breed plants in which this characteristic of storage is predominant: the fat grains of modern wheat are proof of the success of this work.

The third type of carbohydrate has many names, none of which is entirely satisfactory. It is called dietary fibre, although it is not always fibrous; unavailable carbohydrate, although some of it is available to digestion in man; and roughage, although it is not rough! Generally, it is found in the supporting structures of the plant, such as the cell walls of seeds. The most common examples are cellulose, which is in the cell walls of plants and is the material from which paper is made; pectin in fruits, which is the material which makes jam set and is non-fibrous; and lignin, which is woody. To a varying degree, these materials are resistant to the action of digestive juices and pass through the small intestine unchanged.

When we talk about carbohydrates, therefore, we are talking about three quite different classes of food, the sugars, the starches, and the dietary fibre. Each has different characteristics:

sugar is harmful, starch forms the main item in your diet in terms of amount, and dietary fibre helps your bowel to function normally. The rest of this chapter examines the role played by these three carbohydrates in a normal diet.

Do we need carbohydrate?

'Need' is a highly emotive word, used in advertising to sell all kinds of non-essential products, including certain kinds of food. We are told that we 'need' some sort of crunchy breakfast cereal for energy, we 'need' Blogg's meat pies for body-building, we 'need' malted milk for night starvation. For the nutritionist, the word has a specific meaning: if a certain component of food is essential for some process in the body and if that component cannot be made by the body but has to be obtained from food, you are said to 'need' it. Thus, when a nutritionist (as opposed to an advertising man) says that you *need* a certain food, he means that you will die if you don't have it. This is almost certainly *not* true for carbohydrate.

I have to say 'almost' certainly because rigid experiments which exclude carbohydrates from the diet for long periods of time are not practicable in man. However, it has been shown that other mammals (rats, for example) can live in perfect health on protein and fat, without any carbohydrate added. Also, some groups of humans live in good health with a very low consumption of carbohydrate; for example, eskimos have to live almost entirely on meat because plants do not thrive in deep snow. So it seems that perfect health can be maintained on a diet containing hardly any carbohydrate. The energy in these cases is derived from protein and fat.

Although carbohydrate is not essential, the diet in poor countries may contain up to 90 per cent. The reason for the preponderance of this food is that it is palatable, cheap, and easy to grow. Its cheapness was reflected in the old English country custom of serving Yorkshire pudding at the start of the meal, filling up the family stomach before moving on to the more expensive meat course. A similar old custom in Oxfordshire is described by Flora Thompson in her delightful book *Lark Rise:*

On ordinary days, the pudding would be a roly-poly containing fruit, currants or jam; but it still appeared as a first course, the idea being that it took the edge off the appetite. At the big feast there would be no sweet pudding, for that could be had any day, and who wanted sweet things when there was plenty of meat to be had!

Today, in our society, such stringent economies are not practised and we have tended gradually to reduce the amount of starch we eat (although the amount of sugar has increased). Instead, we eat more animal protein and more fat. The first is expensive and unnecessary, the second may do us harm. Recently nutritionists have suggested that a return to a higher proportion of starch in the diet would be a major factor in improving the nutrition of people in affluent countries. In fact in 1976 a committee set up by the American government gave this as the most desirable nutritional change which Americans should make and in 1978 the Department of Health in Britain published similar advice. This advice, together with the other changes suggested to improve the diet, are the subject of the last chapter of this book.

Does too much carbohydrate do you any harm?

Of the three types of carbohydrate, starch and dietary fibre do you no harm (although too much starch will make you fat, as will too much of any food). The other carbohydrate, sugar, is not harmless. Too much sugar is bad for you.

Some examples of different sugars were given earlier but for most people the sugar that is eaten in the greatest quantity is ordinary white sugar. Brown sugar is simply unwashed white sugar; the only difference is the presence of dirt and possibly traces of minerals such as iron. Some people think that it tastes nicer than white sugar but everything said in this section about the harmful effects of sugar applies equally to brown and white sugar. Honey contains various sugars, mostly fructose and glucose, and traces of other substances. The glucose is as harmful as ordinary sugar. The fructose may not be harmful, but experiments on fructose have not been done, so no definite statement can be made about it. It is therefore possible that honey may be marginally less bad for you than sugar, but consumption of large quantities will still have harmful effects because of the glucose it contains.

In the last hundred years the world consumption of sugar has increased enormously, this change overshadowing all other dietary changes which have occurred. Primitive man ate no sugar at all, except that which was present in fruit, and the occasional honeycomb that he was able to scavenge from wild bees. When sugar cane and sugar beet were discovered, commercial cultivation of these crops soon began. In 1850 the production of sugar was 1½ million tons for the whole world, which meant an average consumption of 1·5 kilograms (3 lb) per head per year. By 1970 it had risen to 70 million tonnes, and the average world consumption was then over 20 kilograms (45 lb) per head per year. The figures for Britain are worse, the average Englishman eating 1 kilogram (2 lb) of sugar per week.

Does this do any harm? The first thing it does is to rot your teeth. There is now abundant evidence that sugar causes tooth decay (see Chapter 17).

The nutritionist Professor John Yudkin thinks that it may have other harmful effects; his book *Pure, White and Deadly* states the case. He feels, for example, that the evidence implicating sugar as one of the causes of heart disease is stronger than the evidence implicating fats. He also suggests that a high sugar consumption contributes to the increased incidence of many other diseases including diabetes, chronic indigestion, eye disease, skin disease, and cancer. The evidence Yudkin produces to substantiate these claims is not always convincing; indeed, such evidence is very hard to obtain in man and may never be available: at the present time Yudkin's views seem a little extreme, but his book is well worth reading.

It is difficult to summarize this very contentious subject, and I have discussed it again in chapters on tooth decay, obesity, and heart disease. We do not need sugar; it contains no additional nutrients and therefore fills the diet with 'empty' calories. There is no doubt that it is wise to limit your intake, if only to protect your teeth. This means cutting down on cakes, biscuits, sweets, chocolate, puddings, and soft drinks. It does *not* mean that an occasional bar of chocolate or a serving of pudding will kill you!

Bread, the staff of life

The principal carbohydrate grown in any community is called the staple. The choice of staple will be decided by such factors as the type of soil, the climate, and custom. The staple today in affluent countries is most commonly wheat; it is grown extensively in Russia, India, Argentina, Canada, the United States, and Australia: wherever there is a temperate climate and the soil is good. Rye and oats are grown where the climate is cold and both will survive on fairly poor soil; rye used to be the staple in many Northern European countries but it is being replaced by wheat. Rice is the staple for more people than any other single grain; it grows in damp, tropical climates, being a mud plant and needing a very high rainfall. Maize is hardy and grows easily; it is the 'poor man's staple' in hot dry climates and is cultivated in South America, Africa, and some parts of India and Egypt. Potatoes were the staple in parts of Russia and Ireland. The potato famines of Ireland and the locust plagues in Africa and Asia illustrate how a crop pest can be a disaster to a community relying exclusively on one staple food.

It is very difficult to persuade a community to change its staple food, as many nutritionists have discovered when distributing food to undernourished people. Stories are told of rice-eating Indians dying from starvation while the granaries were full of American wheat which they would not touch, and there are many other examples of the same stubborn refusal to change the diet. In case you should feel complacent, and dismiss this as a quirk of behaviour only to be expected in other people, try to imagine your own reaction if you came down to breakfast and found, not your usual toast, but a dish of rice to go with your marmalade; or if you were offered boiled rice with your hamburger instead of French fries. All men are creatures of habit, and nowhere is this more evident than in their implaccable attachment to their staple food.

Where the staple is wheat, this is usually made into some form of bread. Not all cereals will make bread. Wheat can be made into bread because it contains a protein called gluten which is sticky and which allows the bread to hold its shape when it rises. Rye contains this protein in smaller amounts and can be made into bread, but none of the other cereal crops (maize, barley, rice) can be prepared in this way.

Owing to a tremendous amount of what the Americans would call 'bad press', bread has been very much frowned upon as an item of diet. Firstly, it is supposed to make you fat. This is true of any food if taken in excess of your energy requirement: too much bread *will* make you fat, but so will too much chicken, too much steak, too much yogurt, so why single out bread? Secondly, it is supposed to contain no nutritious substance. This is absolute nonsense. Bread contains a wide variety of nutrients and is almost a complete diet on its own. Five hundred grams (1 lb) of wholemeal flour made into bread would cover your nutritional requirements for one day except vitamin C and vitamin A. Putting a man on bread and water may break his spirit but it does no damage to his health; if vitamins A and C are added, he can live indefinitely on his rations.

There are many different varieties of bread and those people interested will find Elizabeth David's delightful book on the subject very entertaining and full of information. From the dietary point of view, it is important to distinguish between white bread, which is made from flour which has had all the outer husk and the germ removed; brown bread, which covers many types, but by law is allowed to be white bread dyed with caramel colouring; and wholemeal bread. Wholemeal bread is made from 100 per cent extraction flour, that is flour that retains all the outer husk and germ that is present in the full wheat. It has more fibre than white bread and this is a nutritional advantage. It also has marginally more protein and B-group vitamins. The latter differences are only important if you are relying on wheat for all your protein and vitamins. If bread forms part of a mixed diet, the advantage of eating wholemeal bread over white bread is related only to its greater content of fibre. Many authorities have advised that in the diet of affluent countries, replacement of some meat with bread (white or brown), would improve health (see page 40).

What is dietary fibre?

Dietary fibre consists of the carbohydrate which forms the supporting structures in plants. The term 'roughage' was previously used to describe approximately the same thing. It occurs only in plant foods, and not in animal food. It is therefore present in all grains or cereals, like wheat, rice, and oats, and in vegetables and fruit, but is absent from milk, cheese, butter, meat, and eggs. Foods high in dietary fibre are wholemeal bread or any wholegrain food like rolled oats or brown rice; fibrous vegetables such as potatoes, peas, beans, cabbage, celery; fibrous fruits like apples, pears, oranges; and any nuts.

In affluent countries we eat less dietary fibre than we used to. It is frequently removed by the food processers, hence sugar, white flour, and fruit juice contain none, although the foods from which they originate had a high fibre content. The increase in our diet of meat also contributes to our low-fibre diet.

Fibre is not attacked by the digestive juices in the small intestine and is only partially broken down in the large bowel in humans; it therefore contains little available energy for man: so its inclusion in your diet will not make you fat. The bulk foods eaten by slimmers to fill their stomachs and prevent them feeling hungry are often commercially prepared forms of dietary fibre, usually pure cellulose (cell walls).

There are some animals which can, and do, obtain energy from fibre. The fibre is not digested by the action of their own digestive juices, but by means of bacteria which live in the animal's bowel. The bacteria are able to break down the cellulose to various useful products which can be absorbed into the blood-stream. When a cow sits 'chewing the cud', she is shifting grass from one stomach to the next, first breaking it up with her teeth in order to make it more available for bacterial action. When you 'gut' a rabbit, the large segmented piece of gut which dwarfs all the rest of the intestinal structures is the caecum: this is the blind sac in which bacterial digestion of fibre takes place. (There is a small vestigial remainder of the caecum in man, called the appendix.) Since the rabbit and the cow live on grass, which has a very high fibre content in the form of cellulose, it is a great advantage to them to be able to obtain energy from the cellulose, with the help of the bacteria in their gut.

In humans there is a large population of bacteria present in the colon, or large bowel, and a little breakdown of fibre takes place there. Incidentally, it is the bacterial breakdown of fibre which produces some of the 'wind' in the colon; cows and rabbits produce a great deal, and a man changing to a high-fibre diet may notice a rise in intestinal noise levels!

Constipation

Although dietary fibre has only a small nutritive value in man in the sense that it contributes very little energy, no vitamins, and no minerals, it does play a role in the maintenance of health. This role is to facilitate emptying the large bowel.

Dietary fibre has this effect because fibre itself is not absorbed from the intestine and therefore contributes to the bulk of the contents. In addition, it absorbs five to thirty times its own volume of water, increasing the bulk even more. The increased bulk stretches the colon, and since stretch is the normal stimulus which produces emptying, the colon empties more easily. The dietary fibre contained in wholegrain cereal has a greater effect than that contained in fruit.

Constipation is not a disease that kills, but it can cause a great deal of discomfort and distress. It is best defined as a *difficulty* in emptying the bowel; if it is defined on the basis of *frequency* of emptying the bowel, a normal frequency has to be defined and this is not easy. Some healthy people empty their bowels twice a day; others, equally healthy, do so only once every few days with no ill effects. The person who is constipated is therefore the one who has to strain and push, producing hard, pellet-like faeces or stools. His W.C. is often well stocked with books and his medicine cabinet is full of patent remedies. He worries about the effects of the retained faeces; the worry gives him a headache, which he ascribes to the poisons being absorbed from his unemptied bowel. His rectum bleeds and itches from the haemorrhoids he has produced by straining. His friends and maybe even his doctor think that his problem is unimportant (who wants to sympathize over a man's inadequacies on the loo?). Meanwhile the quacks and patent-medicine pedlars make a fortune out of him. A sorry state of affairs!

The solution is: eat more dietary fibre! Almost every single case of constipation can be cured by increasing the fibre in the diet by eating more fruit, vegetables, and particularly more wholegrain cereal. It is not known how much fibre should be included in the ideal diet, but to quote a recent article in the *British Medical Journal:* 'For the moment there is something to be said for the simple view that if a man decides to take all his plant foods in unrefined form, nature itself will ensure that his intake of fibre is right'.

If you are constipated and don't like fruit or vegetables or wholemeal bread, then buy some bran (preferably one without added sugar) and eat 2 heaped tablespoonfuls a day. It can be eaten with milk, or sprinkled or incorporated into any dish such as soups or stews, it will not affect the taste and is not destroyed by cooking. The effect on your bowel habits should be apparent in about two days, and by the end of the week you can throw away the books in the W.C. and the medicines in the cabinet.

The other thing you have to do is to drink plenty of fluids because the bran is much more effective if it is swollen with water. In fact, in some people the diet already contains sufficient bran, but not enough fluid, and lack of fluids alone may be responsible for constipation. Many sufferers report that they are cured by several glasses of water a day.

The great advantage of using bran to cure constipation is that there are no side-effects. Many purgative drugs, even those derived from plants, are very harsh (cascara, senna, and castor oil); they produce spasms in the intestine which are painful, or they are irritant and produce diarrhoea. Also they make the intestine unresponsive to the normal stimulus of stretch, so you have to go on taking them in bigger and bigger doses. Then in the end they don't work at all, and you are back again straining. Bran is absolutely safe, and is particularly useful during pregnancy and in old age, two situations in which constipation is often a big problem.

6 Fats

What are fats?

There is no difficulty in recognizing the 'visible' fats in food; these are butter, lard, and the fat on meat; oil from various vegetables; and margarine which may come from either animal or vegetable sources. Other foods contain what might be termed 'invisible' fat; for example, cream, milk, chocolate, nuts, and cheese.

As a society becomes affluent its consumption of animal fat rises and so does the incidence of cardio-vascular disease. Ancel Keyes, the American medical scientist, thought these two changes might be related and his research has received a great deal of publicity, introducing most of us to the term 'polyunsaturated fats'.

The fat molecule is based on glycerol, which has a shape like a capital letter E. To each of the three prongs of the letter E is attached a long molecule called a fatty acid and it is the fatty acids which can be saturated or unsaturated. A fatty acid consists of a long chain of carbon atoms, up to thirty-five of them, each one bonded by a chemical bond to the carbon atom on either side of it, rather like a chain of people holding hands. A carbon atom, however, has four bonds, and its situation in the chain thus leaves it with two spare ones. These join on to hydrogen atoms, and if, all along the chain, every spare carbon bond is holding a hydrogen atom, the fatty acid is said to be saturated. If there is one carbon in the chain with a spare bond with no hydrogen attached, the fatty acid is unsaturated; if there is more than one spare bond, the fatty acid is polyunsaturated.

Polyunsaturated fats are therefore fats which are not quite full of hydrogen. They occur in plants rather than animals, and they tend to be liquid rather than solid. Thus vegetable fats are usually oils (peanut oil, maize oil, olive oil), and can be collected from plants by squeezing them, while animal fat has to be melted out. When hydrogen is added to an unsaturated fat like peanut oil, it will attach itself to carbon by the spare bonds, forming a saturated fat which is solid. (This is how margarine is made – see page 51.)

Cholesterol is usually classified with the fats, although it is not a fat, having a rather complicated structure unrelated to glycerol. It is worth special mention because its presence in the blood has been used as an indication of the degree of risk from heart disease. The only common food rich in cholesterol is eggs; small amounts are found in meat, and there is none in plants. The human body also makes its own cholesterol, and it has been suggested that the amount it makes may be reduced if poly-unsaturated fats are used in the diet instead of saturated ones (see Chapter 16).

Do we need fats?

In nutritional terms (that is, will we die without them), fats differ from carbohydrates: animals do need them to stay healthy. This was first shown in an experiment on rats in which a group of rats was kept on an artificial diet made up of carbohydrate and pro-tein, fat having been completely excluded. The rats stopped growing; they also developed a scaly skin on their tails. If a small quantity of vegetable oil was added to the diet, the rats started growing again and the scaly skin disappeared. The vegetable oil was then separated into its components, which were added to the diet one at a time, and it was discovered that two specific un-saturated fatty acids, linoleic fatty acid and linolenic fatty acid, are essential to health; they cannot be synthesized in the body and must be provided in the diet. These two fatty acids are present in vegetables but hardly at all in animal fat. The best source for linoleic acid is vegetable seed oils (corn oil, sunflower-seed oil, etc.). Green leaves are now recognized as an important source of linolenic acid: 'Eat up your greens' may well be good nutritional advice on account of their fatty acid content rather than their vitamin content.

Cases of fatty acid deficiency have rarely been reported in humans. There is one report of a man who had lost all but 60 centimetres of his bowel through surgery and had to be fed intravenously: it is very difficult to include fats in intravenous fluids and he developed symptoms of fatty acid deficiency. The rarity of cases in humans suggests that most diets contain adequate amounts.

A second function of fats is related to the fat-soluble vitamins (A, D, E, and K). Since these are found only in fats, a fatfree diet would contain none of them and the risk of vitamin deficiency would arise (see Chapters 9 and 10).

In addition to these two nutritional functions, fats play another essential role in metabolism: that of an energy store. Plants tend to store energy in the form of carbohydrate, usually starch; large amounts are accumulated and the plant grows larger and heavier. Animals store some carbohydrate in the form of glycogen in the muscles and liver; however, every gram of glycogen contributes only 17 kJ (4 kcal), and in addition has to be stored with four to five times its own weight of water. Too much energy stored in this way would make the animal very heavy, no problem for a pumpkin or a potato, but difficult for animals since they have to move around. Fats, on the other hand, are a highly concentrated source of energy, every gram containing 39 kJ (9 kcal). In addition, they do not need to be stored with accompanying water. For one week's activity, glycogen storage would increase your weight by 20 kilograms (40 lb), fat only by 2 to 3 kilograms (5 lb). You can pack enough fat in the bags under your eyes to play a football match!

This capacity to store energy as fat was of great advantage to primitive man who ate at irregular intervals, perhaps when he killed an animal. The excess food eaten at such a feast was turned into fat (it does not matter whether the food is carbohydrate, fat, or protein; it can be all turned into fat), and this fat was stored around the body in the fat (or adipose) tissue until it was needed.

The ability to store fat, inherited from his ancestors, still has important advantages for modern man. The fat store is used for energy between meals, especially if he is exercising. It is an important store in a lactating woman, laid down during pregnancy and available subsequently to help provide the increased energy necessary for milk production. It may also be an important store during a long infective illness, when the appetite is depressed

and the energy need increased due to a high body temperature.
Fat therefore provides a personal, portable larder enabling
survival for long periods without food. It is yours alone, you can
hardly be expected to share it by inviting people to take a bite out
of your bottom! It is this ability to store fat, however, which is
the basis of obesity and for most men in a modern affluent
society it is more of a problem than an advantage.

The storage of fat does have other benefits which are not
strictly nutritional. Firstly, fat stored under the skin insulates
against cold. Again, this has less relevance in modern society
where this function is served by clothing and adequate heating,
although it may explain why women tend to survive exposure
better than men since women store more fat under the skin.
Secondly, stored fat turns angles into curves, making people more
attractive to look at, not to mention touch: who wants to fondle a
skeleton? Julius Caesar even felt menaced by the presence of thin
people.

> Let me have men around me that are fat,
> Sleek-headed men, and such as sleep o'nights.
> Yon Cassius has a lean and hungry look;
> He thinks too much. Such men are dangerous.

Lastly, when considering the advantages of fat there are two
groups of people who find fat useful in their diets simply because
it *is* such a concentrated source of energy. The first group com-
prises those people with a very high energy expenditure, such as
heavy labourers, ballet dancers, and athletes in training. These
people may need up to 22,000 kJ (6,000 kcal) per day, which is
twice as much as the normal requirement. If they could not get
some of it from fat they would be defeated by the sheer bulk of
food they would have to consume. The second group is people
who fast. If you belong to a religious faith which holds days of
fasting or if you know you are not going to get a meal for twenty-
four hours for any other reason, it will help if you make your
'last meal' a very fatty one.

How much fat should we eat?

The high-energy content of fat causes problems in an affluent
society: it is easy to eat too much! There is enough energy
for a whole day in 250 grams ($\frac{1}{2}$ lb) of butter. Also, there is

some evidence that if you eat a lot of animal fats (the saturated ones) you may stand a higher risk of getting heart disease. These harmful effects of fat are discussed in the chapters on obesity and heart disease.

Fat, however, occupies a special place in the cuisine of almost all civilizations and is sorely missed if it is absent. The absolute minimum requirement for satisfaction in this respect seems to be that one-fifth of the food should be fat. Most rich countries eat far more than this: up to 45 per cent of the diet may be fat. In Britain during the war fat was reduced to 33 per cent, and although this was more than enough to maintain good health the reduction was regarded as severe privation and caused much discontent.

In general, if you live in an affluent society you are probably eating too much fat. It may be wise to cut this down and to make a particular effort to reduce your intake of animal fat (see Chapter 22).

The margarine story

Margarine can be made in two ways. The first method uses mutton fat, which is very cheap, and colours and flavours it to resemble butter. The second method uses vegetable oil, and solidifies it by pumping hydrogen into it. Never has an advance in food technology caused such controversy! Wherever margarine has been introduced it has been a political football; for two decades the medical profession has argued about it; even the pronunciation of the word causes argument!

The political controversy dates back to the beginning of the century, when the introduction of a palatable margarine caused great concern to the dairy farmers and there was much political lobbying to have a quota imposed on its manufacture. This lobbying still goes on, sometimes with humour, as in Australia in 1974 when stickers appeared in the back windows of cars claiming that 'butter eaters make better lovers', but more often in deadly seriousness, with claims that the economy of the country will collapse if unrestricted manufacture of margarine is allowed. The lobbying is frequently successful; at various times in most countries the colouring or flavouring of margarine has been prohibited and quotas have been imposed on its manufacture.

The medical side of the story is argued with similar passion. The butter-lovers claimed that butter is a 'natural' food containing 'natural' goodness, better for you than 'artificial' margarine; they apparently feel that a cow is a more natural object than a peanut or a sheep. Then along came the saturated-fats-give-you-heart-disease story and immediately the margarine manufacturers swung into action. The advertising was vigorous, implying that butter travelled direct from the mouth to the coronary arteries, but that margarine eaters would live for ever. This argument ignored the fact that a high proportion of margarine is coloured animal fat, or vegetable fat saturated by the addition of hydrogen and therefore *not* polyunsaturated. Modern methods now use a carefully controlled addition of hydrogen to vegetable oil, producing the polyunsaturated margarines.

What to do? If you are a normal healthy person who does not eat a lot of butter (say, not more than 250 grams (8 oz) per week) or meat (say, not more than four times a week) eat whichever suits your taste and your purse. Margarine is probably a more reliable source of vitamins A and D, which are added to it by law, while butter suffers from seasonal variations in vitamin content.

If, however, you are a high-risk cardiac patient (see Chapter 16 on cardiac disease), then it is worth replacing butter in your diet with margarine which is polyunsaturated. Read the label carefully first to make sure it is polyunsaturated; the price is a good indication since most polyunsaturated margarines cost the same as butter. If you just adore butter and loathe margarine, eat butter and cut down on other animal fats, such as meat, cream, and cheese.

7 Proteins

We come now to the proteins. The word is derived from the Greek word meaning primary, reflecting the primary role played by proteins in many basic biological processes. In nutrition they have always occupied a special place, although sometimes this exalted reputation has led to their wasteful and incorrect use in situations as diverse as starvation, preparation for war, and athletic training.

What are proteins?

For fats and carbohydrates, the major nutritional function is energy supply. This is not so for proteins, whose role is to provide the fabric of the body, by supplying the building blocks for growth and repair.

The basic building blocks are *amino acids*. Twenty of these are found in animals and plants. Each one has its own structure, but all have one feature in common: at one end of the molecule is a chemical group containing nitrogen and hydrogen – the amino group. The amino group cannot be synthesized by animals, only by plants, which are able to use nitrates from the soil. (Some bacteria are actually able to use the nitrogen from the air and incorporate it into their amino acids, proving that some organisms *can* live on air!)

Proteins are formed from chains of amino acids, rather as words are formed from letters of the alphabet, except that the sequences in proteins are longer; for example, insulin contains 51 amino acids, haemoglobin contains 580. Much as the order of letters is important when making a word, so the order of amino acids is important when making protein. Just one amino acid out of order can change the protein; for example, patients with sickle cell anaemia have haemoglobin molecules which differ from normal by only one amino acid out of 580; this tiny difference changes the haemoglobin, and the patient is anaemic.

It is this specificity of proteins which is at the root of their special biological role. A great variety of proteins can be made from twenty amino acids and each organism has its own specific proteins; a peanut has different proteins from a pig, an oak tree from a man. In less major ways, one man has different proteins from another man, so no two men are exactly alike. A great deal of the machinery of the body is devoted to making proteins with the exact amino acid sequences peculiar to the organism and in passing on these sequences to the offspring.

Clearly, since man cannot make the amino group he must get amino acids from his food. During the process of digestion the proteins in the food are broken down to their constituent amino acids in the gut. The amino acids are then absorbed and reassembled into different proteins specific for man. The main organ for this reassembly is the liver, although all the cells of the body carry out protein synthesis to some extent.

Amino acids therefore join that group of molecules which we need not to break down for energy but to play their role in metabolism as themselves. However, unlike the other members of this select group (fatty acids, vitamins, and certain minerals) the amounts of amino acids we need are measured in grams rather than milligrams and this is why protein foods have received such emphasis in programmes to correct undernutrition of all kinds. This question is discussed elsewhere (see, for example, Chapters 4 and 14). First let us look at protein requirements in the normal healthy man.

How much protein do we need?

Human beings need amino acids, in some quantity, all through their lives. Even in a healthy fully grown adult, tissues are being broken down continuously; for example, the lining of the small intestine is renewed every two days and the flakes of skin which collect on the legs consist of dead skin which has to be replaced. In addition to this maintenance, new proteins are being built in any situation in which growth is occurring: that is, in children and in pregnant and lactating women. Also, during an operation or illness, body proteins are broken down rapidly and burnt for energy, and during convalescence they have to be built up again. For all this protein building, amino acids have to be obtained from food.

The most recent figures suggest that 50 grams (1·6 oz) of protein per day is sufficient for a healthy man to keep his tissues in repair. There is much argument about this figure, and healthy communities with a lower intake of protein have been reported. Some authorities quote 30 grams per day as sufficient.

These figures are calculated for dry weight of protein; most protein foods as purchased contain water and other food components. A piece of beef, for example, is 80 per cent water and also contains fat. Here are ten protein foods and alongside each one is the amount (as purchased) that you would need daily if that one food was your sole source of protein (the amounts are calculated on the basis of a need for 50 grams per day).

Lean meat	250 grams (8 oz)
Milk	1·5 litres (3 pints)
Eggs	8
Fish	500 grams (1 lb)
Cheese (Cheddar)	250 grams (8 oz)
Soy beans (dry)	90 grams (3 oz)
Wholemeal flour	500 grams (1 lb)
Peanuts	180 grams (6 oz)
Potatoes	2·5 kilograms (5 lb)

Most diets contain several of these foods, so the amounts should be adjusted accordingly; for example, if you eat a quarter of a large loaf of bread you have already eaten a third of your daily requirement. These daily amounts may not be sufficient for a pregnant or lactating woman or a convalescent patient; such people should eat a third as much again. Very small children need less, but by about 11 years of age a child's requirements are approximately the same as an adult's, that is he needs the amounts shown above.

Is too much protein bad for you?

Most diets in affluent countries contain at least twice the necessary amount of protein, much more than is needed to replace or even build new body tissue. This will do no harm, the body simply burns up the excess protein to provide energy, or turns it into fat and stores it. However, if you are trying to live frugally it might be worth while looking at the amount of protein you eat and, if it is excessive, replacing some of it with cheaper carbohydrate.

Complementary proteins

Although man cannot synthesize the amino group, he does have the metabolic machinery to change some amino acids into others, so if he is short of a particular one he may be able to make it from another which is there in excess. There are eight amino acids, however, which cannot be made by man from other amino acids; these are called the *essential amino acids*. When planning a diet, it is necessary not only to provide a sufficient quantity of protein, but also a sufficient quality; this means the inclusion of all eight of the essential amino acids in approximately the right proportions. A deficiency of just one essential amino acid stops the production of any protein containing that particular one.

Not all foods contain the essential amino acids in the correct proportions for man. Wheat, for example, contains only small quantities of the essential amino acid lysine. Meat and pulses have only low quantities of the amino acids which contain sulphur (methionine and cysteine). The amino acid present in a food in the lowest concentration is the limiting factor in the usefulness of a particular protein. When that one runs out, the rest of the amino acids are turned into fat or burnt for energy, as the body has no way to store them.

This problem is overcome if more of the limiting amino acid is supplied from another protein food. For example, if you were eating only wheat as your source of protein, the deficiency of lysine would mean that a large part of the amino acids in the wheat were wasted. If you supplied food rich in lysine along with the wheat, these amino acids could be used and the available amino acids in the wheat would therefore be increased. Protein foods can therefore be *complementary* to each other. There are two important examples of the importance of this in the diet.

The first concerns meat. Meat, although low in methionine and cysteine, is very rich in all the other esssential amino acids. It can therefore act as a complementary protein food. A small amount of meat added, say, to cereal will make large quantities of cereal amino acids available. This property of meat as a 'spreader' of protein is utilized in many of the great peasant dishes of the world:

Meat with wheat	Spaghetti bolognese
	Stew with dumplings
	Roast beef with Yorkshire pudding
Meat with potatoes	Shepherd's pie
	Lancashire hot-pot
	Fish and chips
Meat with rice	Paella
	Risotto
	Dolmades
	Chinese rice dishes
Meat with oats	Haggis

The second example concerns grain (cereal) and beans (pulses). These two groups of food act as complementary proteins to each other. Cereal is low in lysine but rich in methionine and cysteine; the pulses (like meat) are the opposite. A combination of beans and cereal is therefore rich in available amino acids. Such dishes as lentil stew with dumplings or bread make good sense nutritionally, and the humble baked beans on toast are as nutritious as a piece of roast beef!

The agricultural policy of a country should recognize these complementary properties of proteins; thus the best use of land involves growing cereal as a main crop and pulses as a secondary crop. Those who are planning a diet for a group, whether a family or an institution, are able to economize by reducing the quantity of meat and increasing cereal sources of protein. For people on vegetarian diets, the complementary value of proteins has special importance.

Can you be healthy on a vegetarian diet?

The simple answer to this question is yes. But there are qualifications, and if you want to be a vegetarian for religious, ethical, or financial reasons, it's as well to know the traps.

The range of essential amino acids in some vegetable foods is less complete than in animal foods. This is not always true:

soy beans, potatoes, and rice have a good range but, as already
mentioned, wheat and some beans are deficient. Therefore, if you
rely solely on plant foods as your source of protein, make your
diet as varied as possible to avoid these gaps. In particular, eat
cereal in combination with beans (at the same meal) and include
soy beans, rice (unpolished), or potatoes in your diet every day.

If you follow these rules, you will be just as healthy on a
vegetarian diet as on a diet with meat; maybe even healthier,
because you are eating less fat and more fibre!

Food allergies

Some people come out in spots if they eat lobster or strawberries
or various other foods, and a few suffer more distressing symptoms such as painful abdominal cramp, diarrhoea and vomiting,
or distress in breathing. Such symptoms may be produced by a
food allergy. The subject becomes sensitive to a particular protein in a food, and when he eats that protein an allergic reaction
is produced and may cause any of the symptoms described.

Identifying the harmful food is not always easy. If the symptoms occur immediately, it may be obvious which food is the
culprit, but sometimes symptoms do not occur for several hours.
Skin tests, in which the protein is injected under the skin to see
whether it produces a weal, produce many false negative and
false positive results, so these tests cannot be relied on to identify
the food responsible. A mistaken identification can lead to the
avoidance of a perfectly harmless food and cases have been
reported in which the diet has become unbalanced because a wide
range of foods is being avoided.

When the symptoms occur in babies after drinking cow's
milk, expert advice is necessary because milk forms the whole diet
of a baby and an adequate substitute has to be found; goat's milk
or an extract of soy bean are sometimes prescribed. In adults, if
the allergy is to an exotic food such as strawberries or lobster,
I'm afraid the simplest answer is: stop eating it! If the allergy is
to a common food like eggs or milk, it creates a problem because
so many meals contain these foods. Food allergies of this kind are
not common in adults as most people grow out of them as they
get older.

8 Alcohol

The energy to sustain life is obtained from food in the form of fat, carbohydrate, and protein. There is, however, a fourth source of energy available to man: alcohol. Alcohol is a single chemical substance, ethanol; it contains carbon, oxygen, and hydrogen, as sugars do. In fact alcohol is made from sugar by the action of yeast, this process being known as fermentation. In the human body alcohol is broken down to acetaldehyde, then to acetate, then it can either be used for energy, or it can be converted into fat and stored.

As well as providing energy, alcohol has a further property not possessed by other foodstuffs: it exerts a potent depressant action on the brain and nervous system. Paradoxically, this effect is first seen as an elevation in mood, because the first parts of the brain to be depressed are inhibitory centres and alcohol may therefore have a releasing effect on the personality. As the concentration rises, however, other centres of the brain are depressed; complex functions like speech and walking are affected, then coma may follow and death may occur if the dose is high enough. In this chapter only the nutritional significance of alcohol will be discussed; the pharmacological effects, and the psychological problem, of alcoholism are not discussed except where they are relevant to nutrition.

It is very difficult to quote figures for alcohol and energy content for various drinks because of variations in both the brand of drink and the amount poured. When figures *are* quoted, I have used the following standards:

Spirits: one single (or small)
   whisky, gin, brandy, etc. $\frac{1}{6}$ gill (22 ml)

Sherry, port, vermouth	No statutory size
	'Small' is usually 2 oz (60 ml)
	'Large' is usually 3½ oz (100 ml)
Wine (a glass of white or red)	No statutory size; usually 4 oz (110 ml)

Note: these are pub measures. At home, you or your host will almost certainly pour more than these amounts.

Nutritional value

All alcoholic drinks are made by the action of yeast on sugar. The sources of the sugar and the yeast vary, giving rise to different types of drinks. There are four main types: beer, table wine, fortified wine, and spirits (in increasing order of alcoholic strength).

Beer is made by allowing barley to germinate and then by roasting it to break down some of its starch to sugar, then allowing the roasted barley to ferment with yeast. Finally, hops are added for the bitter flavour. The alcoholic content of beer varies a great deal from 3 per cent in Britain to 10 per cent in some Australian and German beers. Where figures for beer are quoted in this chapter, they refer to the weak variety with 3 per cent alcohol.

Table wines (claret, hock, Moselle, champagne, and many other varieties) are manufactured from fruit, usually grapes, which often have their own yeasts, and which also contain their own sugar. Whether the wine is red or white has no bearing on its alcoholic content, the colour depends on the type of grape used and whether the skin is left in during fermentation. Table wines have a maximum content of alcohol of about 14 per cent (at this concentration the yeast dies), usually they have 9–10 per cent.

Fortified wines (port, sherry, vermouth, Madeira) are made by adding alcohol to table wine and are therefore stronger. Port and sherry, for example, contain 15 to 20 per cent alcohol.

Spirits are made by fermentation of various cereals and vegetables; then they are distilled so that much of the water is removed and a very strong alcoholic drink is obtained. Thus whisky, gin, brandy, rum, and vodka normally contain about 40 per cent alcohol, and overproof samples contain even more. Neat spirits may make the mucosal lining of your stomach and colon very sore and indeed may even make them bleed (see page 63).

One gram of alcohol contains 30 kJ (7 kcal) of energy. The following figures will give you an approximate idea of the energy content of the *alcohol* contained in various drinks:

0·25 litres (½ pint) beer	220 kJ (50 kcal)
1 glass wine	290 kJ (70 kcal)
1 small sherry	250 kJ (60 kcal)
1 single whisky (gin, brandy, vodka)	220 kJ (50 kcal)

Alcoholic drinks contain other sources of energy besides alcohol, mainly in the form of sugar. This contribution to the energy value is normally small. It may add another 50 per cent in the case of beer, but sweet wine, for example, has an energy content only 20 per cent greater than dry wine.

Apart from alcohol, and small amounts of sugar, alcoholic drinks contain nothing of nutritive value. There may be traces of vitamins; also some minerals, depending on the method of production, but these are irrelevant in the over-all nutrition of the individual. Alcoholic drinks, like sugar, represent empty calories and a person relying on alcohol for a large part of his energy intake often suffers from malnutrition. He may be eating too little protein, and he frequently shows signs of vitamin deficiency. This has caused confusion in determining the harmful effects of alcohol, since these may be due not to the alcohol itself, but to a concurrent vitamin deficiency. For example, an alcoholic may develop muscular weakness in the legs which makes walking difficult, and pins-and-needles sensations in the skin. These are signs of nerve degeneration and are due not to alcohol, but to lack of vitamin B_1; a high proportion of his energy is being obtained from alcohol, and there is too little food to provide an adequate supply of the vitamin. Any person who relies on alcohol for more than one-quarter (3,000 kJ or 750 kcal) of his total energy intake will run the risk of dietary insufficiencies, particularly of vitamins.

Harmful effects and hangovers

There are of course several harmful effects of excessive drinking which are due directly to the action of alcohol and are not nutritional in origin. These include damage to the liver, brain, and heart. All of these are due to the direct poisoning effect of high concentrations of alcohol on the tissues concerned. Little is known about the mechanism by which alcohol produces these harmful effects, but the liver damage has been much studied.

One 'binge' will produce liver damage which can be seen microscopically as fatty infiltration of liver cells, and measured biochemically as changes in enzyme levels in the blood; these changes disappear over the following few days. However, if the binge is repeated often, the damage becomes permanent and cirrhosis of the liver may occur. Not all heavy drinkers develop cirrhosis, but in any community there is a very close relationship between the incidence of the disease and the average level of alcohol consumption.

As far as can be determined, the liver damage is produced by alcohol itself, and not by any other ingredients of the drink; therefore there is no support for the suggestion that certain drinks are worse than others. For example, one often hears it said that spirits are more likely than beer to harm your liver. This is not true: the total alcohol consumed is what matters, therefore a pint of beer is as dangerous as a double scotch in this respect.

How much alcohol can you drink without running the risk of cirrhosis? The figures for safe levels of alcohol intake for an individual are not available, one of the problems being that individuals vary greatly in their susceptibility to the disease. There is much argument; some authorities suggest that two drinks a day may produce cirrhosis in susceptible individuals. This seems rather overcautious; up to four drinks a day is probably safe, but intakes greater than this are certainly accompanied by increased risk.

Another unpleasant, although not nearly so dangerous, side-effect of alcohol is the 'hangover'. If you haven't ever had a hangover it may be difficult to appreciate how awful it is! There is a feeling of malaise, characterized by gastro-intestinal upsets, such as diarrhoea or general queasiness; headache; and fatigue;

and all the rest of the world seems to be very bright and noisy. These symptoms are due to two effects: firstly, the damage done by the alcohol, secondly, the effects of other poisons present in alcoholic drinks.

Some of the damage done by alcohol involves the cells lining the gut. High concentrations cause marked irritation, to the stomach and especially to the colon; after a hefty binge there is often bleeding. The symptoms may include abdominal pain, lack of appetite, nausea, and diarrhoea. This damage can be avoided to some extent by diluting the alcohol with food. Fortunately, since the lining of the gut replaces itself every couple of days, the damage heals.

In addition to this damage to the gut, alcohol also increases urine flow to amounts over and above the volume of fluid taken, so that over all it has a dehydrating effect. This effect of alcohol lasts all the time that there is alcohol in the blood, therefore it cannot be counteracted by drinking more water while you are still drinking alcohol. What you must do is to drink copious water after the event: before going to bed if you stopped drinking early at the party; otherwise next morning as soon as you get up.

There are other toxic substances in alcoholic drinks which contribute to the hangover. Firstly, there are substances similar in structure to alcohol and called congeners. These are broken down by the liver more slowly than alcohol is, so they hang around longer. Secondly, histamine is present in some alcoholic drinks; this substance is well known to produce headache.

Some drinks have more congeners and histamine than others. In an experiment volunteers were given equivalent amounts of alcohol in eight different drinks and their hangover symptoms were recorded. Hangovers were most distressing after brandy, then in decreasing order of severity came red wine, rum, whisky, white wine, gin, vodka, and pure alcohol. In fact, after vodka and pure alcohol, dehydration (thirst) was the only symptom noted. Therefore, if you want to minimize the risk of a hangover, it may be worth avoiding red wine and brandy and sticking to vodka or gin.

Both congeners and histamine tend to be present in higher concentrations in new wine, and both tend to disappear as wine matures. Therefore if you drink older wine it may produce a less distressing hangover: an advantage counteracted by its effect on your pocket!

All sorts of hangover cures have been tried over the years and everyone has his own favourite – a sure sign that all of them are fairly ineffective! Recently some experiments in London have suggested that fructose (fruit sugar) and large doses of ascorbic acid (vitamin C) may increase the rate at which the liver metabolizes alcohol. If you want to increase the speed of clearance of alcohol from your body, take two glasses of orange juice (vitamin C) flavoured with a couple of dessertspoonfuls of honey (fructose) before you go to bed. A mild antacid may help the gastrointestinal symptoms. Next morning if you still feel ghastly repeat the treatment and make the usual resolution: not so much next time, you're getting too old to take it!

The blood alcohol level

When an alcoholic drink is swallowed, absorption of the alcohol into the bloodstream begins from the stomach. This is unusual; most foods are not absorbed until they pass from the stomach into the intestine, and then only when they have been broken down to simple molecules. Alcohol is different, its rapid absorption is due to two factors. Firstly, it does not have to be broken down by digestive juices; it is absorbed unchanged. Secondly, it mixes readily with fats, and since all cell walls are fatty, this speeds absorption.

If the stomach is empty, absorption is even more rapid and alcohol will start entering the blood only a minute or two after the drink is swallowed. Drinks taken with or after solid food will be more slowly absorbed. It used to be thought that drinking milk or oil before drinking alcohol would delay absorption, but this does not seem to be so. In an experiment in New Zealand, some happy volunteers drank a pint of milk followed by two double whiskies; then the next night they drank the whisky without drinking milk first. Measurements of their blood alcohol showed that the milk did nothing to delay the absorption of alcohol.

As alcohol is absorbed from the alimentary canal, the liver begins to break it down at the rate of about 7 grams per hour. This rate of breakdown is constant and continues until all the alcohol has gone. The level of the blood alcohol thus depends on how quickly alcohol is entering the bloodstream; if you drink more alcohol than the liver can handle, your blood alcohol will go up. To put it another way, every hour you can drink one half pint of beer, one small glass of wine, one single scotch, or one sherry, and your liver will destroy the alcohol as fast as it is absorbed from the gut. At this rate of drinking you will not be affected by the alcohol, you will stay sober.

At faster rates of drinking, alcohol will accumulate in your blood while it is waiting to be broken down by the liver. The maximum permitted blood alcohol level for driving varies from 50 to 100 mg/100 ml. All sorts of factors will determine how many drinks are necessary to achieve this level, but as a rough guide, if you are average size and have an empty stomach, four pints of beer, or five glasses of wine, or five double scotches, drunk over a couple of hours, would put you well in the danger zone.

The slow rate of metabolism of alcohol means that it can take all night to metabolize the drinks from one evening. Say, for instance, you go out to dinner and you have two sherries, four glasses of wine, and two brandies (an evening at the pub with six pints of beer will give you the same amount). Your liver will only just have finished dealing with the sherry by the time you go home! The rest of the drink will put you over the legal limit for driving a car, and when you wake up at 7 a.m. next morning your liver will be still patiently working away on the brandies! If you drink more than the amount given in the above example, you will be getting up next morning still under the influence of alcohol, and if you drink double the amount stated your blood level will still be high enough for you to be charged with driving under the influence while on your way to work!

9 Vitamin deficiencies

What are vitamins?

A vitamin is a substance which is necessary in very small quantities for some metabolic process in the body, but which the body cannot manufacture; it therefore has to be provided in the food. These substances have been the subject of intensive study over the past fifty years, and their chemical formulae are now known. The vitamins known to be required by man are:

Vitamin A	retinol
Vitamin B group	thiamine (B_1)
	riboflavine (B_2)
	folic acid
	pyridoxine (B_6)
	cyancobalamin (B_{12})
Vitamin C	ascorbic acid
Vitamin D	calciferol
Vitamin E	tocopherol
Vitamin K	naphthoquinone

Nutritionists usually classify vitamins into those soluble in fat, and therefore found in fats (A, D, E, and K), and those soluble in water (B and C). All the vitamins can be manufactured in the laboratory and there is absolutely no difference between these 'synthetic' vitamins and the 'natural' vitamins found in food. Each will have the same action in your body, each is equally good for you, or in large doses equally bad for you.

There is so much information available about vitamins, and so much interest in them, that I have divided the subject into two chapters. In this chapter there is an account of the vitamin deficiencies. In the following chapter I have concentrated on the practical aspects of vitamins in an affluent society: which foods contain them, the effect on them of cooking, whether vitamin pills pick you up, and whether large doses will do you any harm.

The story of scurvy

In 1497 Vasco da Gama sailed around the Cape of Good Hope. It was a marvellous feat of exploration; nevertheless it killed two-thirds of those on board. It must have been a terrible voyage, one man having to do the work of two, then three; and that man hardly able to drag himself around. These sailors had scurvy because they had no fresh fruit or vegetables, and they died through lack of vitamin C. At that time no one knew the reason, and for the next four hundred years sailors went on dying on long sea voyages in the same way.

Looking back on those four hundred years, there were many clues. For example, in 1535 the French explorer Cartier put ashore in Newfoundland and one of his crew, who had been sick, returned from a visit to the natives apparently cured. Cartier questioned the man and discovered he had drunk a concoction brewed from the pine needles of the spruce tree. When this infusion was given to the rest of the sailors, they all recovered from their scurvy. The event went unnoticed.

Over two hundred years later a Scottish naval surgeon, Lind, carried out a trial on the ship *Salisbury*. He took twelve patients, all very sick with scurvy and near to death, and he divided them into pairs, each pair receiving one of the following additions to their diet:

> A quart of cider a day
> 25 drops of sulphuric acid
> 2 spoonsful of vinegar
> Half a pint of sea water
> 2 oranges and a lemon
> A pill of garlic, mustard, and myrrh

Lind reported that the two sailors eating oranges and lemons recovered so quickly that they were fit for duty at the end of six days (one was so well recovered that he was appointed to nurse the rest of the sick!). None of the other 'cures' worked. Lind published his results in 1753 in a 'Treatise on Scurvy'. A few explorers noted the results; Cook's exploration of the Pacific probably owed its success to the fact that he seized every opportunity to put into shore and supply his men with fresh food. But throughout the nineteenth century, three hundred years after Cartier and the pine needles and a hundred years after the publication of Lind's treatise, sailors continued to die.

Even when the importance of fresh food was recognized, it was not always possible to make adequate provision. In his journals of his expedition to the South Pole, Scott speaks of the 'dreaded scurvy'. When he and his companions set out on the final trek, however, they carried no source of vitamin C. Convenient tablets were not available because the pure vitamin had not been isolated, fresh fruit and vegetables were too heavy to carry, and sprouting seeds (beans or cress) would probably not have germinated in the cold. Since they were away from the base camp for several weeks and in addition were doing hard physical work, which increases the need for vitamin C, they were almost certainly deficient in the vitamin. It is probable that the tragic deaths which followed would not have occurred had the party not been weakened by scurvy.

How much of each vitamin do we need?

The answer to this question is not known with any certainty because of the difficulty of doing the appropriate experiments. First an artificial diet has to be prepared which contains no vitamins. Usually, purified starch or sugar is used as the carbohydrate, purified corn oil as the fat, and the protein is added in the form of amino acids as pure chemicals. All the vitamins not being studied are then added, producing a diet which theoretically is adequate in every respect except for the vitamin under investigation. This diet may have to be fed to the animal for several months before signs of deficiency develop because some vitamins are stored in the body in quantities sufficient to last several months. When signs of deficiency do develop, the missing vitamin has to be added to the diet in measured amounts until an amount is discovered which just maintains health.

These are long, tedious, and expensive experiments. To discover the dietary requirements of the rat for vitamin A, for example, might take a thousand rats and occupy two people full time for two years, if all went well. But the final snag is that the results may not be applicable to humans because their require-ments differ. Man shares his requirement for vitamin C, for example, with only the monkeys, the guinea pig, and the South American bulbul bird! Consequently the experiments have to be carried out in humans and this means that volunteers have to be found. Imagine the advertisement for volunteers for such experiments:

WANTED

Volunteers for scientific experiment. Subjects will have to eat an arti-ficial diet containing no natural foods. They will have to live in an institution during the experiment, which may last 1–2 years. At the end of the experiment they may feel very ill.

Clearly one is not going to be overwhelmed by volunteers! Such experiments involve constant medical examination of the subjects as well as meticulous preparation and continual analysis of the diet. Finally, there is a risk involved. One of the first such experiments was carried out in 1770 by the Scottish physician William Stark, using himself as a volunteer; he died of the scurvy he induced.

For these reasons, the scientific data are sparse. I have described the problem in some detail so that the next time you read on the food packet that the contents will supply you with your daily requirements of a certain vitamin, you may view the statement with a healthy scepticism because no one knows exactly what your daily requirements are.

What are the vitamin deficiency diseases?

In some cases the exact role played by a vitamin in metabolism is known; for example, vitamin A is the precursor of a pigment in the eye which enables you to see at night, vitamin D is necessary for calcium absorption from the gut and so is important in the development of teeth and bones, vitamin B_1 is an essential factor in the process of breaking down carbohydrate to provide energy.

In many other cases the physiological role of a vitamin is not understood. Even if we do not understand exactly what a vitamin does in the body, however, the symptoms of vitamin deficiency have been well studied. The absence of a particular vitamin in the diet produces a deficiency disease. Many of these diseases are accompanied by general lethargy, weakness, and susceptibility to infection. There are, however, some specific symptoms related to each vitamin.

Lack of vitamin A produces night blindness, due to a lack of pigment in the retina. The other symptoms of vitamin A deficiency are related to changes which occur in all the epithelial, or surface, cells. These cells undergo excessive multiplication and become heaped up on one another, producing a scaly skin and horny plugs in the sweat glands. These epithelial changes in the cornea of the eye produce blindness if the disease is not treated. Vitamin A deficiency is almost unknown in affluent countries, but there are many areas of South East Asia, the Middle East, Africa, and America where a large number of children between the ages of 1 and 5 years go blind due to lack of vitamin A. Of all the nutritional diseases, this one perhaps illustrates best the difficulty of correction: a few pence per child would pay for enough vitamin to prevent blindness but distribution of the vitamin has proved an insuperable obstacle to eradication of the disease.

Lack of vitamin B produces a variety of symptoms because there are many members of this group of vitamins. Two well-known deficiency diseases are beriberi and pernicious anaemia. Lack of vitamin B_1 produces beriberi, a disease associated with weakness and general lassitude. In severe cases there may be marked retention of fluid, causing the typical pot-belly of beriberi found in communities subsisting on polished rice. There may also be degeneration of nerves so that paralysis and lack of sensation occur. Lack of vitamin B_{12} produces pernicious anaemia, called pernicious (or wicked) because sufferers always died from it, until it was found that eating vast quantities of raw liver cured the disease. When vitamin B_{12} was discovered, pernicious anaemia was treated by an injection of the vitamin every few weeks (no doubt a great relief to those eating the raw liver!).

Lack of vitamin C produces scurvy. The first symptom is a feeling of fatigue and listlessness. Later the collagen which helps to bind cells together breaks down and bleeding occurs into joints, under the skin, and in the gums. The sufferer may have little spots on the skin of his feet and legs where haemorrhage has occurred, and widespread bruising is produced by the slightest injury.

Lack of vitamin D causes rickets: bones and teeth do not develop properly due to the lack of calcium, which is not absorbed from the intestine if there is no vitamin D. The effects vary according to the age of the child. In South Africa, for example, very early infancy is the time when vitamin D is most likely to be in short supply since mother's milk is a poor source, especially if the mother is deficient. The bones of the skull do not close, and the rib joints form knobs which used to be called 'rickety rosary'. When the infant starts crawling around in the sunshine he makes his own vitamin D (see page 76) and the symptoms disappear. In low-income families in Scotland the picture is different. Infant feeding with the help of an advanced social welfare programme is usually adequate because of free vitamin supplements. When the baby starts feeding with the family, the supply of the vitamin becomes inadequate and there is too little sun to help him out. The limb bones fail to form properly and do not support his weight, giving rise to the knock knees and bow-legs of rickets, and spinal deformities may also occur.

Lack of vitamin E has not been reported in human adults. However, there is some evidence that it may occur in babies, particularly premature babies, and that the vitamin may be useful in the treatment of various problems in the newborn, including anaemia and breathing difficulties. These effects are currently being studied.

Lack of vitamin K causes bleeding, due to the failure of the blood to clot. Normally, as soon as bleeding occurs on injury, the blood starts to coagulate and form a clot which stops further bleeding. Many factors in the blood are necessary if coagulation is to occur normally and vitamin K is necessary for the formation of prothrombin, one of these factors. Therefore if you lack vitamin K, your blood will not clot and any injury will produce excessive bleeding.

In the early 1940s in Canada cattle fed on spoiled clover developed a tendency to bleed. It was shown that dicoumarol, a substance present in the clover, antagonized the action of vitamin K. This discovery led to the production of the rodent poison Rat Sak: the mice or rats are given wheat which has been soaked in dicoumarol and later die from haemorrhage. Dicoumarol and drugs related to it are used in patients suffering from thrombosis (a disease in which a blood clot blocks a vital artery); the use of these drugs is known as anticoagulant therapy.

Do vitamin deficiency diseases occur in affluent societies?

Some vitamin deficiency diseases are seen even in affluent societies. Examples are scurvy (vitamin C), rickets (vitamin D), and beriberi (vitamin B_1).

The group in the community most susceptible to scurvy is the elderly on a low income and within this group the men seem to fare worse than the women. These old men come to hospital outpatients' departments with symptoms of scurvy. They usually come in the spring because their main source of vitamin C is potatoes, which have a high vitamin C content when harvested but tend to lose it on storage over the winter. As soon as the new potatoes appear in the shops, the number of old men with scurvy decreases.

Anyone not eating carefully cooked vegetables or fresh fruit risks getting the disease. If you are one of those who is too busy to be bothered much with food, you may be short of vitamin C; eat some fresh fruit or vegetables every day or drink some fresh orange juice. If this is too much trouble buy some ascorbic acid tablets from the chemist, they are quite cheap. The strength to buy is 30 mg; take one every day; alternatively, a single one-gram tablet once a month is just as effective.

Another disease sometimes seen is rickets. Cases have been reported in children of poor families living in the northern hemisphere in big cities, where the hours of daylight are short, and any sunlight which would allow them to make vitamin D in their skin is filtered through the smog. A second susceptible group is any migrant population, for example, in Britain and Australia. These children are protected from the sun by clothing or by the dark pigment of their skins (this did not matter in their own country, with almost unlimited sunshine). Also the family diet tends to include few dairy products, being based on vegetable oils, which do not contain vitamin D. Children are affected more than adults by a shortage of vitamin D, because their need for the vitamin for bone formation is proportionately greater than that of an adult.

Another disease seen in affluent societies is beriberi in alcoholics. The causes are complex and not entirely understood, but one of the major reasons is that an alcoholic eats hardly any food, since he obtains the greater part of his energy in the form of alcohol. Alcohol, although a source of energy, contains no other nutrients; it is 'empty' calories. Consequently, alcoholics run the risk of suffering from dietary deficiencies of all kinds, and the damage to the nerves caused by lack of vitamin B_1 is the most common.

Every time a human being moves out of his natural, familiar environment, the risk of vitamin deficiency occurs. In a familiar environment, experience leads to the choice of an adequate diet from the foods available; if the environment is changed, the man will not know how to compensate for the dietary inadequacies which may arise. Examples are: sailors on long voyages; migrant populations; children in northern industrial cities covered by a blanket of smog; and even old widowed men, who, removed from the familiar environment of the family, are unable to choose an adequate diet for themselves. The nutritionist can identify these groups, make them aware of the gaps in the diet, and teach them how to fill them with cheap, readily available local produce.

10 Vitamins: practical considerations

Which foods contain vitamins?

Vitamin A occurs naturally only in animal fat, the richest sources being milk, butter, cheese, eggs, and liver, particularly the liver of certain fish like cod and halibut. Vegetable oils contain none at all, but margarine which is made from vegetable oil is required by law to have vitamins A and D added to it in some countries.

Strictly speaking man does not need to obtain vitamin A from his diet since he can make it from *carotene*, a yellow pigment found in certain plants. In those parts of the world where no animal products are eaten, carotene is the sole source of vitamin A, while in the normal mixed European diet about half of the vitamin A comes from this source. Carotene is found in all highly coloured plants such as carrots, the outer dark-green leaves of cabbage and spinach, and tomatoes.

The following foods each provide sufficient vitamin A for a healthy adult for one day:

Halibut-liver oil	1 drop
Cod-liver oil	small teaspoonful
Butter or margarine	100 grams (3 oz)
Milk	2 litres (4 pints)
Cheese	120 grams (4 oz)
Liver	100 grams (3 oz)
Carrots	100 grams (3 oz)
Dark-green leafy vegetables	100 grams (3 oz)
Orange juice	4 litres (8 pints)

Vitamin B is the name given to a group of substances (thiamine, riboflavine, pyridoxine, folic acid, and vitamin B_{12}) which have been classed together because they tend to occur together in the same foods, except for vitamin B_{12} (see next paragraph). These vitamins are present in small quantities in all animal foods. However, by far the richest source is seeds, such as peas, beans, lentils, and wholegrain cereals. The vitamins are present in the germ of the seed, and are largely removed if the grain is milled. This does not matter if a mixed diet is eaten, but where the main source of energy is a single staple milling may result in a diet deficient in vitamin B. Thus in rice-eating countries the consumption of polished (milled) rice leads to the appearance of beriberi. The B-group vitamins are also present in yeast, although enthusiasts of yeast and yeast extract (Marmite, Vegemite) should note that they would have to eat 30 grams (1 oz) of yeast or yeast extract per day if that was their sole source of vitamin B_1.

Vitamin B_{12} is unique among vitamins as it has to be obtained from animal sources, so that really strict vegetarians who do not eat milk, eggs, or cheese would be expected to suffer from pernicious anaemia. They usually do not, a fact which has puzzled nutritionists for many years. They obtain the minute quantities necessary from sources which are unknown but which almost certainly include yeasts, moulds, and bacteria. These organisms all make vitamin B_{12} and vegetarians may thus obtain supplies of the vitamin from contaminated food, or from water which has run off soils containing these organisms. Less hygienic food preparation will increase the supply; for example, village cooking by Hindus in India probably allows inclusion of vitamin B_{12} from these sources.

It is almost impossible to suffer from vitamin B deficiency on a mixed diet. Here are some foods which are good sources of these vitamins:

> All wholemeal cereal
> Pulses
> Meat and dairy products
> Yeast, yeast extract
> Bran
> Drippings from roast meat

Vitamin C, or ascorbic acid, has a limited distribution and is susceptible to damage by handling and cooking. In any Western diet it is the most likely vitamin to be present in deficient quantities. The main sources of vitamin C are citrus fruits, currants, berries, green vegetables, potatoes, and growing seeds such as cress and bean sprouts. All of these should be fresh, and if cooked they should be cooked as quickly as possible (see page 78). The following foods each contain sufficient vitamin C for a healthy adult for one day:

Potatoes	250 grams (8 oz)
Oranges	1 orange or 1 small glass of juice
Cabbage	100 grams (3 oz)
Bean sprouts	1 cupful
Blackcurrant syrup	1 glass of diluted drink

Vitamin D is not a vitamin in the true sense because it can be manufactured by the body. The production of vitamin D occurs in the skin, where derivatives of cholesterol are acted on by sunlight to produce vitamin D. Hence if you get enough sunshine on your skin you don't need any vitamin D in the diet at all. If, however, you are deprived of sunshine (far northern climates) and if the limited sunlight available is prevented from reaching the skin (too many clothes, too much smog, or a dark skin), you will have to obtain all your vitamin D from food. The following foods are rich in vitamin D:

> Cheese
> Eggs
> Butter and margarine
> Cod-liver or halibut-liver oil (danger, see page 81)

Vitamin E The richest sources of this vitamin are vegetable oils. Wheatgerm oil, sunflower-seed oil, and safflower oil have a particularly high content of vitamin E. Since some margarine is made out of vegetable oils, this represents an important source in any diet containing margarine. Many other foods contain vitamin E: it is present in moderate amounts in eggs, butter, wholemeal cereals, and broccoli.

Vitamin E deficiency has not been reported in man, so that it appears that all known diets contain a sufficient quantity.

Vitamin K The main source of this vitamin is green leafy

vegetables that are fresh, such as broccoli, cabbage, lettuce, and spinach. Ox liver is also a good source.

Vitamin K is also produced by bacterial action on food and by the bacteria that live in the large bowel of man. It is probable that this latter source is sufficient and that man needs none in his diet. Certainly no deficiency has been reported in adults, so either dietary sources or production in the gut are adequate for all known requirements.

Does cooking destroy vitamins?

The most unstable vitamin is vitamin C, which starts to break down when it is exposed to air. There is an enzyme in plants which speeds the destruction of this vitamin. In the intact plant the vitamin and the enzyme are stored apart but cutting or bruising the plant lets the two come into contact and increases the loss of vitamin, so that loss begins as soon as the plant is harvested. Then, because vitamin C is water soluble, it will be leached out of the vegetables into cooking or washing water. Lastly, heat will speed up the destruction, especially if the cooking water is alkaline as it is when bicarbonate of soda is added. It is amazing that any vitamin C survives at all, and indeed very little does if the foods are overcooked or kept warm for long periods of time, as they might be in a canteen. However, by taking certain precautions, up to 80 per cent of the vitamin survives. I have summarized these precautions at the end of this section.

In view of these losses of vitamin C in cooking, it has been suggested that we eat our vegetables raw. Whether you would get more vitamin C this way is debatable. The vitamin is inside the cells in the vegetables. The cell walls are not digested, and relatively few are broken by chewing, so it is possible that some of the vitamin passes through the gut locked inside its vegetable cells. Eat raw vegetables if you like them, but don't assume that you are getting much more vitamin C than from carefully cooked vegetables.

Vitamin B_1 (thiamine) is the other vitamin which suffers a significant loss in food preparation. It is fairly resistant to destruction by heat, especially in an acid medium (for instance, baking bread with yeast, which produces acid, does not destroy it). However, it will dissolve in water, particularly if bicarbonate is added. This loss is extremely important in communities living largely on rice, which is washed first and then cooked in water, and which may lose all its vitamin B_1 before being eaten. The use of very small quantities of water for washing and cooking the rice may be a critical measure in preventing beriberi in such communities.

In summary, the vitamins lost in cooking are vitamins B_1 and C. When cooking fruit and vegetables, this loss will be far less if the following precautions are taken:

1. Cook as soon as possible after picking.
2. Cook in as little water as possible.
3. Exclude oxygen by boiling the water first to drive off the oxygen, and by using a small pan with a tight lid.
4. Put the vegetables into boiling water to kill the enzyme which destroys vitamin C.
5. Do not use bicarbonate.
6. Cook for as short a time as possible.

Do vitamin pills pick you up?

There are certain people who need extra vitamins, for instance pregnant women and babies not being breast-fed; these are discussed in Chapters 12 and 13. There are other situations in which the requirement for a particular vitamin is raised; for example, after a long infective illness or a major operation the patient needs extra vitamin C. In such situations a doctor may prescribe extra vitamins; taking them will improve health, and the doctor's advice should be followed.

Lots of perfectly healthy people, however, buy vitamin pills. Anxious mothers give them to growing children. Aspiring athletes eat them to make themselves run faster. Tired business men eat them to make themselves less tired. Wealthy women have injections of vitamins 'for their nerves'. Every year vast sums of money are spent on vitamins, a tribute to the success of a vigorous and constant advertising campaign.

If you are on a mixed diet which includes the foods described earlier in this chapter you do not need vitamin pills. You will obtain enough vitamins from your food and enough is enough; eating more will not make you any healthier. Despite the claims of the manufacturers, extra vitamins will not improve your temper, your energy, your nerves, your resistance to disease, or your sexual performance. Except in the special circumstances described, money spent on vitamin pills is money wasted.

Will very large doses of vitamins cure diseases?

There have been claims that very large doses of vitamins will cure certain diseases. These claims are much more dangerous than the claim that vitamin pills will pep you up. Firstly, they may prevent sick people from obtaining medical advice and thus delay effective treatment; secondly, large doses of some vitamins are poisonous, and may even kill you.

The only effective use of large doses of vitamins is in the treatment of *specific deficiency diseases*. In other words, large doses of vitamin C will cure scurvy, large doses of vitamin D will cure rickets, and so on. There is absolutely no evidence at the moment that any single disease, apart from vitamin deficiency, is helped by large doses of any vitamin. Thousands of claims have been made, but three have won especial popularity: vitamins for schizophrenia, vitamin C for colds, and vitamin E for just about everything.

The vitamins-for-schizophrenia claim may have particularly tragic consequences. Large doses of vitamins have been used in an attempt to treat the disease; in fact the term 'vitamin mega-therapy' was coined to describe the treatment. Hundreds of hopeful patients were put on the treatment, some recovered, but many more got worse because they were removed from their current care, counselling, and support. Then careful trials were made, and it was shown that the therapy was useless.

How can such mistakes be made? The layman, confused by the arguments of the so-called experts, is entitled to ask the question. Firstly, schizophrenia is difficult to diagnose and some patients put on the treatment probably did not have the disease. Secondly, the disease sometimes goes into temporary remission without any treatment, and this probably clouded the picture. Thirdly, and most tragic of all, schizophrenia is primarily an incurable disease and desperate relatives unable to accept this fact will clutch at straws. Having clutched at a straw, and spent much money in the process, they are often loath to admit failure and will exaggerate the slightest improvement to justify their decision.

The second example is related to vitamin C. Professor Linus Pauling, who won the Nobel prize for chemistry, has written a book called *Vitamin C and the Common Cold* (1970) in which he claims that the consumption of very large amounts of vitamin C will protect you against colds. He writes very persuasively, arguing that man's natural diet used to contain large quantities of fresh vegetables with correspondingly large amounts of vitamin C and that a return to this level of consumption is a return to the natural state. As a protective measure he suggests you eat 1–2 grams of vitamin C per day (to obtain this amount from natural sources, you would need to eat 40 oranges, 6 kilograms (13 lb) of potatoes, or 4 kilograms (8 lb) of cabbage). Once you catch a cold, the recommended intake is 2–10 grams daily.

Pauling's claims have been tested by many scientific groups. Here is a brief description of one such trial, to give you an idea of the problems involved. The trial was set up to see whether vitamin C would reduce the symptoms of a cold once it had started. Four scientists in Britain studied 1,524 people, recruited from two retail stores, an engineering plant, a large industrial group, a local government office, and the staff of a hospital. Every person was given a bottle of tablets, labelled with a code number. Half of the people received tablets containing vitamin C and the other half had dummy tablets made to look and taste like vitamin C. However, most important in a trial of this nature, neither the subjects nor the people handing out the tablets knew which code numbers represented real vitamin C and which were dummies.

The people in the trial were told to start taking their tablets as soon as they suspected that they were getting a cold, and to continue taking one every six hours. Meanwhile they were to record their symptoms under the following headings: runny nose, muscular aches, days in bed, days off work, and total number of days the cold lasted. Obviously, people's reporting of these various symptoms varied, and one man's idea of how long the cold lasted may be quite different from another's.

At the end of the study, which lasted right through one winter from December to April, the results were collected. No difference was found between the two groups, that is those taking the real vitamin C tablets experienced exactly the same length and degree of symptoms as those taking the dummy tablets. The scientists running the trial therefore concluded that there was no case for recommending vitamin C against the common cold.

Well, that looks fairly conclusive! However, other workers have obtained different results. For example, in 1975 Canadian workers found in a trial involving 2,349 people that large doses of vitamin C taken at the start of a cold *did* reduce the duration and severity of the illness. Conflicting results have also been obtained in trials to see whether vitamin C can prevent colds (rather than cure them).

Pauling's book continued to arouse interest and no doubt many family doctors were besieged with patients asking whether they should take vitamin C. In 1976 the *British Medical Journal* published an editorial comment on the subject which stated that '. . . at present no strong evidence can be found to support the routine prophylactic (preventative) use of ascorbic acid in well nourished people'. In other words, vitamin C will not *prevent* colds. It goes on to say that there is uncertainty about its use as a cure. Taking it once a cold has begun may have a beneficial effect on some people. It also points out that large doses taken for long periods may be harmful.

The third example is vitamin E. Claims have been made that the following conditions are cured by vitamin E: miscarriages, menopausal disturbance, heart disease, sterility, skin disorders, and poor sexual performance. It is also said to improve athletic performance. In fact, not one of these claims is supported when adequate trials are carried out. Vitamin E is not a cure-all; as far as can be seen it is not a cure-anything, and no case of vitamin E deficiency in man has ever been reported.

Having said that vitamin megatherapy does no good, the next question to ask is: does it do any harm? Unfortunately, it does. The fat-soluble vitamins A, D, E, and K are stored in the body (mainly in the liver) and their storage levels can build up, with serious consequences. For example, high levels of vitamin D can produce symptoms such as a headache, lethargy, coma, and even death: this has been observed in children who were the victims of misguided maternal enthusiasm and were given extra halibut-liver oil in the belief that if a little is good for them more is better. Cases of vitamin A toxicity have also been reported in some women taking large quantities of the vitamin for skin complaints. Cases of vitamin E toxicity have not been reported. The water-soluble vitamins (B and C) are not so dangerous. However, an excess of vitamin C acidifies the urine and may cause stones to form in the bladder, so large doses of the vitamin should not be taken.

All this has been said before, and it will be said again. It will make little difference to the consumption of vitamins. People will continue to take vitamin C for colds and sunflower-seed oil for heart attacks, and desperate relatives will continue to try vitamin megatherapy for schizophrenia. Until certain cures are found for the incurable diseases, we shall continue to clutch at straws. Advertising is far more powerful than fact.

11 Minerals and trace elements

All of the food that we eat, both animal and vegetable, comes from the soil, the sea, and the air. During evolution some of the elements that are present in these three parts of the planet became incorporated into metabolic processes and are essential to man. He must obtain these essential elements from his food.

Many elements are necessary in only very small quantities and are present in the body in such low concentrations that it is difficult to measure them; these are the trace elements. Their importance in animal nutrition may have been proven, but whether all of them are essential for the health of man is very difficult to establish. It is possible that in the future their role will be better understood. A nutritional deficiency has never been shown for them in man, so for this reason I am not going to discuss them in any detail. They include the following elements: tin, vanadium, nickel, silicon, aluminium, molybdenum, chromium, selenium, manganese, cobalt, copper, and magnesium.

Other elements have a well-established and much studied role. They are sodium, closely related to the water balance of the body; iron, the mineral of the blood; calcium, the mineral of bone; iodine, the atom which forms part of the molecule of the thyroid hormone; and zinc, which has just stepped on the scene as an element which may be deficient in the diet of some children. All of these are discussed in this chapter. Fluorine, the element which reduces tooth decay, is discussed in Chapter 18.

Sodium

Sodium is the element which, together with chlorine, makes up ordinary table salt. Its presence in the body is regulated very accurately by the hormone aldosterone from the adrenal gland. Its importance is related to the fact that the amount of water held

in the body depends very largely on sodium. You can only
expand the amount of water in your body by increasing the
amount of sodium; conversely, you can reduce it only by
reducing the sodium. This does not mean that a healthy person
can consciously manipulate his water-holding capacity; his
hormones will compensate for anything he does by conserving or
eliminating extra salt. People with various forms of heart failure,
however, often have a disturbed hormonal balance and are
unable to maintain this very fine regulation. This may lead to
oedema (a collection of water in the tissues which produces
swelling), which can sometimes be corrected by a reduced salt
intake. They are often placed on a salt-free diet for this purpose.

Salt is very widely distributed in food, and the body also
conserves salt very well; there is therefore no need to add any salt
to food. Nevertheless people do add salt to food because they
like the taste of it. From Roman times salt has been considered a
valuable item; the word 'salary' is derived from the Latin for salt
because the Roman soldiers used to be paid in salt. Nowadays
salt is very cheap and we can all eat as much as we want to.
However, an excessive amount of salt in the diet may lead to
harmful side-effects.

It is difficult to think of the ubiquitous table salt as being
harmful, but evidence is accumulating that it is. For example,
in communities in which the intake of salt is very high the incidence of heart disease is also high. Also, rats fed on a diet containing extra salt developed high blood pressure while rats fed
the same diet without the salt did not. The experts argue about
the importance of salt in causing heart disease, but since we do
not need added salt, it seems wise to avoid eating heavily salted
foods too often, not to be too heavy handed with the salt shaker
at the table, and not to add too much salt when cooking. The
addition of salt to the food of babies and children has particularly
dangerous consequences because it educates them to a salty taste
early in life and the natural development of this taste means that
by adulthood they will probably be looking for a very high salt
intake. This problem is discussed in Chapter 12.

Do we ever run short of salt in our diet? This is unlikely to
happen for two reasons. Firstly, salt is very widely distributed in
soils and therefore most plant foods contain it; secondly, *all* foods

derived from animals contain salt.

There are, however, some areas of the world in which the soil is deficient in salt. These areas are the large land masses situated away from the sea so that they derive no salt from sea-water spray. Crops grown on such soil contain very little salt and animals that feed on grasses in these areas are salt deficient. The animals conserve salt by excreting urine with hardly any salt in it. In addition, they seem to develop a specific appetite for salt. This was shown by Derek Denton, an Australian scientist, and his colleagues. In the Snowy Mountain regions of Australia, where the soil is very deficient in salt, pegs soaked in various solutions were put into the ground. At night-time the rabbits came out and chewed on the pegs that had been soaked in solutions of sodium salts, like common salt, but ignored pegs soaked in similar-testing solutions which contained no sodium.

Whether humans show a similar specific appetite is hard to prove, since there have rarely been communities where salt deficiency was a problem. Some people claim to feel a 'craving' for salt at various times but it is often difficult to relate this to a time of need. Denton has wondered whether some of the less attractive customs of humans such as cannabalism, or grinding up ancestral bones and eating them, may have their basis in a craving for salt. You are liable to lack salt after copious sweating, or after vomiting; you may hanker after salty foods at these times and this may be the vestige of a specific salt appetite. The dangers of salt in all advanced cultures are related to eating too much rather than to deficiency; for example, a 'fast-food' meal may contain over a teaspoon of salt. Any changes in our diet should be directed at a reduction of this (page 157).

Iodine

Iodine is an essential part of thyroxine, the hormone from the thyroid gland. This hormone has two functions. In infants it is necessary for normal growth and development; infants deprived of iodine do not make enough thyroxine for normal development and are dwarfed physically and retarded mentally. They are known as cretins. In adults thyroxine controls the basal metabolic rate. Adults who are deficient in iodine have a very sluggish metabolism; they feel the cold and tend to put on weight.

Iodine deficiency occurs in those areas where the soil has a low iodine content, because all the produce and the water of such areas contain very little iodine. In such areas there is a large incidence of cretins and the adults often have a goitre, a swelling of the thyroid gland in the neck. The swelling is produced because the growth of the gland is stimulated by pituitary hormones which are secreted in response to the low levels of thyroxine. People with goitre often manage to make enough thyroxine for their needs and show no sign of thyroxine deficiency.

The regions which are deficient in iodine are scattered all over the world: they include mountainous areas such as the Alps, the Himalayas, the Andes, and the Rockies; and alluvial plains such as those of the Great Lakes in North America. In Britain one such area is the Derbyshire peak district; the term 'Derbyshire neck' refers to the goitres frequently seen there. In Australia the island of Tasmania is similarly affected. In an attempt to eradicate the problem it has been suggested that iodine be added to table and cooking salt (iodised salt) but this suggestion has not always been followed by the appropriate authority.

Iodine is widely distributed in many foodstuffs and, if your region has a normal level, you will run no risk of deficiency. If you live in an iodine-deficient area (your doctor or local health authority will be able to tell you) it is wise to buy iodised salt, particularly if you are likely to become pregnant, as it is in the very early stages of the development of the child that iodine deficiency is most dangerous.

Calcium

The human body contains large quantities of calcium, found almost entirely in the bones and teeth. Half of living bone is calcium phosphate, the rest is water and protein; for bone is a living tissue and the store of calcium is constantly turning over. The bones of a child are replaced completely every two years, and even in an adult they change their material every ten years or so.

Many factors control this perpetual removal and replacement of calcium, and nutrition does not normally play an important role. Hormones (the hormones from the parathyroid gland) are the main factors, but mechanical stress also has an important effect. Stress tips the balance in favour of keeping calcium in the bones. Even a healthy man loses calcium if the normal stresses on bone are removed; if he is kept in bed without any exercise he will lose a lot of calcium from the bones and this will have to be replaced when he starts walking around again. Astronauts lose calcium owing to the lack of gravitational forces, which prevents the stress on bones normally produced by their own weight. In the elderly, calcium loss from bones increases and the bones become brittle and easily broken. This is not always prevented by increasing the calcium in the diet; exercise may be a more effective way of treating the problem.

The richest dietary sources of calcium are milk and cheese, with cereal being the next best source. The calcium in cereal may not be as readily available as that in milk because wholegrain cereal contains phytic acid, a substance which strongly binds to calcium and prevents it from being absorbed from the gut. When this effect was first shown at the beginning of the Second World War, the 'national loaf' was being introduced. This bread was made of high-extraction (wholemeal) flour, so to counteract the effect of phytic acid, extra calcium was added to the flour. Although milk is now freely available, and also the importance of the effect of phytic acid has been questioned, flour is still fortified with calcium in many countries. In the absence of vitamin D, no calcium can be absorbed from the food (see page 71).

Obviously the need for calcium is greatest during periods of growth, and pregnant women and growing children need a great deal. These special needs have been described in Chapters 12 and 13. Adults need calcium only to replace that lost in the urine, and a mixed diet will adequately supply these needs; calcium deficiency is seldom seen after growth has ceased.

It has sometimes been suggested that calcium deficiency may be the cause of cracking and splitting finger-nails. There seems to be no evidence for this. A much more likely cause is trauma to the nail; that includes banging it in any way, on a typewriter for example, dipping it in detergent, or bending it. These insults to the nail should be avoided as far as possible. Keeping the nails very long will increase the risk; painting bright nail varnish on them may help by its constant reminder that the nails are there. (Eating gelatine will do no good unless you are lacking the sulphur-containing amino acids contained in meat and pulses, which is highly unlikely.)

A recent observation on heart disease may have some connection with calcium. During the last few years several studies in different countries have shown that the incidence of heart disease is lower in areas where the water is hard. Since the most common cause of water hardness is the presence of calcium salts (present in water drawn from chalky soils) it has been suggested that calcium may have a protective effect against heart disease. No mechanism has been suggested for this effect of hard water, nor has it been demonstrated directly that calcium is responsible. As the scientists are fond of saying, further experiments may produce interesting results. Meanwhile, if you live in a hard-water area, forget the problem of the soap not lathering; it is just possible that you are deriving some benefit from the hard water in terms of a reduced risk of heart disease!

Iron

Iron is part of the haemoglobin in red blood corpuscles. These cells are continually broken down and replaced by new ones. However, the body is very prudent with its iron and the iron from broken-down red blood cells is carefully conserved and used again, so that only small quantities of iron are lost in the urine and sweat.

The absorption of iron from the alimentary canal is a complex process and only a fraction of the iron in the food gets across this barrier into the blood. The absorption is increased if vitamin C is present. Foods which contain the most iron are meat (especially liver) and pulses and cereals. Experiments have shown that iron is absorbed more readily from meat than it is from vegetable sources, so a diet rich in meat is the best nutritional way to treat anaemia. However, meat is expensive and such a programme is not practical in communities of poor resources, where anaemia is most common. The best treatment in these areas is to give iron tablets. Tablets of ferrous sulphate are the cheapest, and the iron is as well absorbed from these as it is from the more expensive iron preparations.

If blood is lost, as in a haemorrhage, an iron deficit is created and has to be restored. Women of child-bearing age lose blood regularly during menstruation and in childbirth and also excrete iron in their milk. Women of this age are therefore susceptible to iron deficiency, which will lead to a low haemoglobin and anaemia. The symptoms are fatigue, breathlessness on exertion, lack of appetite, sleeplessness, and pallor of mucous membranes. The symptoms are insidious and many women who have anaemia adjust their pace of living to allow for it; they work slowly and for short periods.

Even in an affluent society, if you are female and of childbearing age, you may be anaemic. A simple blood test by your doctor will determine this. If you are anaemic and can afford (and enjoy) meat and liver, eat them at least once a day for a few weeks.

If you are a vegetarian, it is difficult (although not impossible) to correct anaemia when eating only plant foods. Orange juice, because of its vitamin C, will greatly enhance the absorption from plant sources. Tablets of ferrous sulphate may also be used. A course of tablets for a month will top up your iron stores and correct any deficiency for several months. Ferrous sulphate may make you constipated, in which case one of the other iron preparations should be used.

Children, because they are increasing their blood volume by growth, also need extra iron. This will be adequately provided by a mixed diet; tiredness and inability to do sustained physical work in children in affluent societies are more likely to be due to boredom and lack of exercise than lack of iron.

Zinc

A great deal of recent work suggests that zinc may be deficient in some human diets. Zinc is important because it is essential to the functioning of many different enzyme systems: over forty were listed in a review published in 1979. These included the enzymes necessary for the synthesis of DNA (desoxyribonucleic acid) and RNA (ribonucleic acid) which are the basic molecules controlling cell division and protein synthesis in all cells in the body. Thus a deficiency of zinc would be expected to have far-reaching results.

Zinc deficiency in humans was first observed on a large scale in adolescents in Iran. The diet of these people consisted largely of unleavened bread, and it was suggested that the fibre and phytic acid content of the bread bound the zinc and prevented its absorption from the bowel. The children were stunted in growth and showed delayed sexual maturity.

Deficiency has since been observed in babies who were fed on cow's milk, and it has been suggested that the reason in these cases is again related to absorption, the zinc in human milk being much more easily absorbed than that in cow's milk. Babies who were deficient again showed stunted growth. Many modern baby formula foods were analysed and found to have insufficient zinc for the growing infant. This has now been corrected.

Zinc deficiency is almost certainly rare in adults, possibly because their needs for zinc are proportionately smaller. The foods which contain the most zinc are oysters, which contain twenty-five times as much as any other food. However, if you don't live on oysters (and who does?) you will also get zinc from meat, cheese, peanuts, and wholegrain cereal.

12 Feeding babies and children

In affluent societies adequate food together with good advice on infant feeding are freely available to most people and the problems of feeding babies and children are associated with too much, rather than too little. There are three particularly common excesses: too much food, too much salt, and too much sugar. These are discussed in this chapter, together with that phenomenon of the affluent society, baby foods. Children do, however, have certain special nutritional requirements which have to be taken into account if there is any shortage of food; these are their proportionately greater needs for Calories, protein, and calcium.

Special needs of children

There are two reasons why a child needs proportionately extra food. Firstly, the basal metabolism of the child is high because of the extra work his body is doing in growth. A newborn baby doubles its birth weight in five months and quadruples it in three years, and although growth then slows down a little, there is a second spurt at 11 years for girls and 13 years for boys. The energy cost of growth is high and the child needs food to cover it. Secondly, a child is much more constantly active than an adult. It has been calculated that the energy spent on movement by a 3-year-old in a normal day would carry an adult up the stairs to the top of the Empire State Building!

The other special needs of the young child are high-quality protein for building the tissue of the body, and calcium for bone growth. Both of these will be covered if the family is eating a mixed diet, but if you want to be especially sure, give the child extra milk. Half a litre (1 pt.) a day provides all the calcium needed and a third of the total protein. Milk is not essential for children's health, however, as long as there are other sources of calcium and protein in the diet.

In any community where food is short, it is important to stress these special needs of the children, because families who do not know about them tend to give the lion's share of the food to the bread-winner. A child of 11 years of age, even though he has reached only half the adult weight, needs a full adult ration of food with respect to total energy and protein, and more than the adult ration of calcium. If he does not get these, his growth will be stunted physically and there is also the possibility that his mental development will be retarded (see Chapter 4).

Too much food

In the United States, in Australia, and in Britain, recent surveys have shown that many children are fat. Obesity is discussed at length in Chapters 2 and 3, but obesity in children merits special discussion, because fat children often make fat adults. The reason is not known, but one recent finding may be relevant. While children are growing, the cells in their fat tissue increase in both size and number, and fat children have been shown to have a greater *number* of fat cells. It is possible that overeating in childhood may leave a legacy of extra fat cells, so that there is the potential for a large amount of fat tissue.

These effects have been demonstrated in rats. Twenty newborn rats were divided so that eighteen were given to one mother to feed and the remaining two, the 'privileged' pair, had a mother to themselves. The privileged pair, getting much more milk than the eighteen who were fighting for eight teats between them, became fat. The fat rats had an increased number of fat cells in their fat tissue, and in addition when all the rats were weaned and allowed to eat what they wanted, the two privileged rats *continued to eat more, and stayed fat*.

This experiment has frequently been interpreted to mean that overfeeding in infancy may lead to the development of eating habits which result in overeating and obesity in later life. But are these findings applicable to humans? How can human babies 'overfeed'?

A baby is not a free agent when it comes to food. He has to take what is offered. It has been shown that bottle-fed babies tend to be heavier than breast-fed babies and the following reasons for this have been suggested. Breast-fed babies suck until they have had enough, then they stop; no one knows how much they have eaten, so no one worries. A bottle-fed baby may leave some milk; if he does, it is in a glass bottle for everyone to see, and mother gets worried and tries to coax him into eating it. Often she succeeds, so the baby eats more than he wants. In another study it was shown that bottle-fed babies generally receive solid food much earlier than breast-fed babies; again, the baby is eating more than he wants to. Finally, when bottles are made up from dried milk powder or a proprietary formula, many mothers add extra powder so that the mixture is richer than the manufacturers planned, and the baby has to eat more just to satisfy his thirst.

Scientific data about rats and population statistics on fat children may convince the nutritionist, but most of us firmly resist the implication that we overfeed our children. One reason for this resistance may be that we are members of a society which tends to relate eating not to hunger, but to family relationships. Look at the following list, and you will see what I mean:

What we say	*What we mean*
He never eats a thing.	He doesn't eat everything I put on his plate.
He's outgrown his strength.	Where's my cuddly baby?
Don't eat that; it'll spoil your dinner.	I've spent all morning preparing dinner and you're jolly well going to eat it.
You've left some of your dinner.	You don't like my cooking.
I've cooked you a new pudding.	I love you.

This last remark sums it all up. In the family situation today, food is inextricably bound up with love. The cook (usually the mother) thinks that if *they* don't eat the food she has prepared it means that *they* don't love her. To discard such attitudes is not easy but if you are the family cook, the following hints may help you to avoid overfeeding your children.

First, let's consider babies. If you bottle-feed your baby, don't force him to finish the bottle. If he is on a proprietary brand of dried food, measure the powder carefully, don't throw in an extra measure for luck, and if the label says a *level* measure don't put in a heaped one; scrape it level with a knife. In addition don't give solid food to a baby too early. In many primitive societies a baby drinks milk and only milk for nine months or longer; in fact, until it has teeth to cope with solid food. It therefore seems sensible to delay solid food. At about six months, start him off on the blander dishes from the family table: a bit of mashed potato, a little egg yolk, so that he gets used to a variety of adult foods.

For older children, the same principles apply. Don't force them to eat. Offer them food, and if they don't want it put it away and let them down from the table; for children, eating is not the social occasion that it is for us and they won't die of starvation before the next meal! Try not to offer alternatives to tempt them, or snacks between meals; they tend to choose the sweetest and thus form tastes which will make them fat later.

It may be as well to conclude by emphasizing something that was said in the chapter on obesity: fat children have been shown to eat less on the whole than thin children. It is often their activity level which is different, and the most effective way to combat obesity is by encouraging your children to be active.

Too much salt

Salt (sodium chloride) is essential to life, but it is not necessary to add salt to the food of babies and children, since natural food contains adequate amounts. The only exception to this rule is when the baby is sweating copiously in hot weather, or when it is vomiting or has diarrhoea, when it may be necessary to give salt together with a lot of liquid to drink to replace that being lost.

It is easy to omit salt when you are preparing the baby's food yourself. However, if you are using prepared baby foods it may be more difficult. Manufacturers of baby foods discovered that their product would not sell unless it contained quite a lot of salt, because the mother tasted the food and if it contained no salt she found it bland and tasteless and searched for a saltier brand. In other words, the food for the baby was being chosen to suit the palate of an adult and these babies had an unnaturally high salt intake in early life. Since there is a gradual increase in salt appetite with age, their salt intake as adults would be very high indeed.

There is evidence that too much salt increases the risk of heart disease. If you prepare food for babies or children, add no salt. If you buy baby food, check the taste and *avoid* the salty ones (most manufacturers are reducing the salt content). For older children, 'take-away' and 'fast' foods are usually heavily salted; do not let these become a major part of the diet.

Too much sugar

The third mistake to avoid in feeding babies and children is too much sugar. The dangers of sugar have been described; it is in the early years that a taste for sugar can be unwisely encouraged.

When a baby is bottle-fed, the cow's milk or other substitute is often sweetened with sugar (sucrose), which is much sweeter than lactose (the sugar found naturally in milk). Thus the baby is accustomed to a sweet taste very early in life. It is better to use lactose instead and many proprietary formula bottle foods do this. You can check the contents on the label.

Many brands of solid baby foods have sugar added to them; even in unlikely meals like chicken livers or brains sugar is often one of the ingredients listed on the label. The reason for such formulation is economic, the addition of sugar being simply a cheap way of adding bulk to the food.

The same traps are there to catch the children as they grow up. Sugar turns up in the most unexpected places: baked beans, tomato soup, and peanut butter are some examples. Breakfast foods are toasted so that some of their starch is broken down into sugar, and some of them even have a sugar frosting added to the individual flakes. Biscuits, cakes, and sweets are thrust at children in magazine, radio, and television advertisements. Well-meaning friends and relatives bring bags of sweets as gifts for the children.

What can one do? While the scientists have produced the evidence, it is the parents who are left with the day-to-day problem of excluding sugar. Babies are easy; just cut sugar right out by breast-feeding or by mixing the formula with lactose, never adding sugar to their solid food, and never, never dipping their dummies (comforters) in sugar or honey. With older children it is much more of a problem. Total exclusion is very difficult in our society; certainly I am incapable of exerting the discipline needed to achieve it in my own family. But a great deal can be accomplished by having no sweet foods (biscuits, cakes, sweets), lying around the house and not cooking dishes where sugar is a main ingredient. For further details see Chapter 18.

Breast-feeding and baby foods

During the first few months of its life, all the nutritional requirements of a baby will be provided if it is breast-fed (assuming that the mother is healthy). There are several nutritional advantages of breast-feeding. The composition of human milk is exactly right for the baby and it is delivered at the right temperature and in the right quantity. The milk passes from 'inside-the-mother' to 'inside-the-baby' with no external contact and is therefore free of germs. The first few feeds contain antibodies (very young babies make none of their own) and this may explain why breast-fed babies are more able to resist infections, and possibly cot-deaths. There may also be emotional advantages deriving from the close physical contact between the mother and baby, especially if the process of breast-feeding gives the mother pleasure, as it usually does. In an affluent society breast-fed babies tend to be less obese than bottle-fed babies. In poor countries breast-fed babies have a higher chance of survival and it also costs far less, an important consideration in these countries (see page 102).

Some mothers, however, cannot breast-feed their babies, and for these babies an alternative has to be found. One of the first alternatives used was cow's milk. A baby with no mother's milk would die, and it must have occurred quite early to primitive man that cow's milk might do instead. Cow's milk differs from human milk in that it contains over twice as much protein and three times as much salt, so it has to be diluted with water. After dilution it contains too little carbohydrate, so sugar is added. Such a mixture makes a satisfactory substitute; the usual formula is 60 millilitres (2 oz) cow's milk, 30 millilitres (1 oz) water, 3·5 grams (one level teaspoonful) sugar. It is easy to see one disadvantage of such a mixture: it is much sweeter than human milk owing to the addition of sugar, and it may encourage a sweet taste in the child as well as damaging teeth as they appear—dental decay has been reported in children at 2 years of age! The remedy is to use lactose (milk sugar) instead.

The next development was the production of the dried food in powdered form. This usually consists of cow's milk which is dried and often modified to be more similar to human milk. When required for use, the only addition necessary is water. The danger with dried preparations is that if they are made up overstrength the baby is receiving an energy and a salt load which is too high. The excess energy content will be converted into fat. The extra salt may be dangerous, not only because of the relationship to heart disease already discussed but on a short-term basis. Salt has to be excreted through the kidneys: if the formula is made up too strong, the infant kidney, which is less efficient than an adult kidney, cannot handle the additional extra salt and the baby may die owing to salt intoxication. The way to avoid this is to make up the feed exactly to the manufacturer's instructions. The most common mistake is to use a heaped measure when the manufacturer's instructions say a level measure.

Encouraged by the enormous success of dried milk formulae for babies, food manufacturers then turned to the older child and a massive menu of foods for toddlers is now available. Used as convenience foods, once or twice a week, these are quite harmless – indeed, they are invaluable to a busy mother. The tinned foods are particularly useful when travelling, as they are sterile. However, proprietary foods have several disadvantages if used all the while. They may contain excessive salt; they may contain unnecessary sugar; and they do not educate the child to eat the normal family diet, particularly with respect to texture, since most baby foods are fairly mushy. This means that when the transition to the family diet is made, the baby may not make it easily. For these reasons, it is better to feed the growing infant at the family table and to save proprietary baby foods for convenience.

For mothers

People should have every sympathy with mothers; they are bombarded by the experts with advice which is likely to be different from year to year. You may be advised to feed your first baby like clockwork, every four hours, and your last whenever he feels like it. They both seem to survive. Have the people telling you what to do ever coped with a hungry baby screaming at 3 a.m. or tried to explain that he's had his ration for this twenty-four hours and an extra feed will make him fat? Or a 2-year-old who is quite happy to sit at the family table and eat the family diet as long as you give him all your attention and don't eat a thing yourself! Or a 10-year-old who won't eat the cabbage, whether you cajole, scream, or deprive her of pudding; she just doesn't want to know about scurvy!

My advice is this. Relax! All children are different. Most grow up to be healthy in spite of all the advice. Try to cut down their sugar. Try not to force them to eat something if they really don't want to, even if it's taken you hours to cook. Feed them more if you feel they are hungry, and if they get fat (your postnatal clinic or doctor will tell you) keep them up an extra half hour and increase their physical activity. Lastly, when you feel worried say firmly to yourself: MOTHER KNOWS BEST, and listen to your intuition. Good luck!

13 Eating during pregnancy and lactation

It has long been recognized that the period during which a woman produces and feeds a child must produce nutritional stress. This is reflected in the old saying 'feeding for two' and in many tribal customs of giving a pregnant woman special titbits from the meal. The nutritional stress, however, can be met easily, providing that the woman goes into pregnancy in good health and that adequate food is available. Problems arise in countries where food is in short supply and the reserves of the woman are therefore low: she has no stores of important minerals like iron and calcium, she carries no fat to give her a reserve of energy; even her own tissue proteins may be depleted. Under these circumstances the extra strain of pregnancy poses a great burden. The developing child takes what it needs and depletes her still further. Malnutrition (unless extremely severe) does not affect fertility, so there is the likelihood that she will become pregnant again before she has recovered any reserves. She is on a downward spiral of depletion. Even in wealthy communities there exist poverty pockets where a combination of poor nutrition and repeated pregnancies have resulted in women producing stunted babies.

In this chapter I will describe the extra nutritional needs of a pregnant woman. Then the needs during lactation are given, together with an account of the unprincipled exploitation of these needs by big business in Third World countries. Finally, a brief note is given on pregnancy sickness and unusual appetites, both problems of minor importance in the over-all picture, but not to the woman who is suffering from them!

Pregnancy

During pregnancy the average weight gain is 12·5 kilograms (28 lb). A third of this weight gain is due to the foetus and the liquid it lies in. Another third is made up of an increase in the weight of the mother's own tissues; the uterus and breasts, for instance, increase in weight by 1·5 kilograms (3 lb) and an extra 1·5 litres (3 pints) of blood are produced. The final third is fat; during a normal pregnancy a woman accumulates 4·5 kilograms (9 lb) of fat which forms an important reserve to be called on during lactation.

Weight is not gained at an even rate throughout the nine months. Over the first twenty weeks about 3·5 kilograms (8 lb) is gained, then the rate speeds up to half a kilogram (1 lb) a week. These are average gains and can vary quite a lot with no danger to health; however, if the weight change differs from these figures by more than 50 per cent a careful search for the cause should be made. Too little gain may indicate inadequate development of the baby; too much indicates either fluid retention or excessive accumulation of fat, neither of which is desirable.

The first need therefore is extra energy. Over the nine months an extra 850 kJ (200 kcal) are needed each day. There is, however, a specific need for protein as well and it is important that some form of high-quality protein should be included in the diet. The distribution of the amino acids in the protein must be such that the correct range is present for new tissue to be built and that means animal protein such as meat, fish, or milk; or soy beans or a combination of cereal and pulses if the woman is on a vegetarian diet.

The third special need is for calcium. During pregnancy twice as much calcium is needed so that the foetus may build bones and teeth. If this is not provided in the mother's diet, the baby does not go short but takes his calcium from the mother's bones and teeth. The old country saying 'for every child a tooth' reflects the fact that the foetus functions as a parasite in this respect! However, the total needs during pregnancy and lactation will not deplete the mother unless she has a poor diet and numerous pregnancies. Milk is the best dietary source of calcium, cereals are second best. Since vitamin D is needed for the absorption of calcium, this needs to be allowed for as well (either adequate sunlight or extra dairy products).

The two other requirements are extra iron and one of the B-group vitamins, folic acid. Both are needed for making the extra blood. The mother's blood volume increases to allow for extra blood to flow through the placenta and nourish the foetus. In addition, the foetus itself is making blood; a newborn baby has about half a litre (1 pint). The over-all increase is up to 2 litres (4 pints), representing a need for about one gram of extra iron (one small nail!). Dietary sources of iron and folic acid are meat, pulses, and whole cereal. If dietary iron is short, again the foetus does not suffer since it uses up the mother's iron stores. In poor communities, where an inadequate diet has reduced maternal iron stores, anaemia is common during pregnancy. Because of this, together with the uncertain absorption of iron, many authorities recommend routine administration of extra iron in tablet form in the last three months of pregnancy. Lack of folic acid also leads to anaemia and again it is sometimes advised that this vitamin should be taken in tablet form in the later stages of pregnancy.

In summary, the extra needs during pregnancy are energy, protein, calcium, iron, and folic acid. In a wealthy community these extra needs will almost certainly be covered by the normal mixed diet. If you are pregnant and want to be especially sure, take a supplement of a pint of milk a day, and iron and folic acid pills in the last three months if your doctor advises it.

Lactation

During lactation the nutritional needs of the mother are greater than they were in pregnancy. Although the baby's growth rate slows a little after birth, he is bigger, so that each increment in size represents a greater amount of tissue being built. Also he is more active than he was in the uterus and all the energy for this movement has to be derived from the mother, via her milk.

An extra 2,100 kJ (500 kcal) are needed per day; this is a considerable amount – equivalent to an extra meal a day. As with pregnancy, there is also a need for high-quality protein as the baby needs amino acids for building his body tissues. In addition extra calcium, iron, and folic acid are needed as they were in pregnancy.

These heavy nutritional demands made by a baby are most economically met by giving the mother extra food, NOT by bottle-feeding the baby. This point needs emphasizing. In recent years the pernicious practice of selling artificial baby foods in Third World countries is a prime example of the way in which nutritional truths can be totally distorted by unscrupulous men.

In his book *The Baby Killer* (War on Want, London, 1974) Mike Muller exposed this activity. The manufacturers of baby foods were sending teams into Third World countries to persuade the mothers that bottle-feeding was better than breast-feeding. Great advertising hoardings were erected which depicted well-dressed plump babies being bottle-fed on commercial baby foods, with the hidden implication that bottle-fed babies and affluence go hand in hand. The selling methods were unprincipled: representatives of the company were dressed as nurses and went to give 'nutritional advice' to the mothers; free samples of commercial baby food were given to the mother in hospital; the hospital received free equipment in exchange for recommending the commercial baby food to its maternity cases. After the first week of use, the mother's milk would dry up, thus establishing a continuous need for the commercial product. The cost of feeding a baby this way is very high. The following figures were quoted for Nigeria; the figures are slightly out of date but the relative differences are the same:

Cost of extra food for a lactating mother	21 pence per week
Cost of cheapest baby food (skimmed milk)	32 pence per week
Cost of commercial baby food	£1.15 per week

In human terms, the cost was the lives of the babies. They died, either from starvation because their families ran out of money to buy food, or from infection because the standards of cleanliness needed for artificial feeding are impossible to maintain in a primitive community. In 1979 a second publication, *The Baby Killer Scandal*, by Andy Chetley, stated that after five years of campaigning against the manufacturers (including Nestlé, who account for over half the market) the situation is almost unchanged. The amount spent in 1978 on commercial baby food in the Third World was £300 million. A small fraction of this money injected into the agricultural system of these countries would have given the mother the extra food she needed to breast-feed her baby and the benefits would still have been there to feed the baby when he was weaned. Thousands of lives would have been saved. Mammon, unfortunately, was too strong.

In affluent communities there is enough food available, although some women do find it difficult to eat sufficient while breast-feeding and they lose weight. Others notice that they can eat as much as they like and put on no weight themselves, which rather pleases them! There is the reserve of fat which was laid down during pregnancy to draw on during lactation; mothers who do not breast-feed should note that they have to get rid of this by other means, e.g. walking 5 kilometres (3 m.) a day or eating only half their normal food for approximately forty days.

Pregnancy sickness and special appetites

Most women, on learning that they are pregnant, are anxious to eat sensibly for their baby but many suffer from nausea and some actually vomit during the first three months of pregnancy. This troublesome symptom may make eating very difficult. There have been many suggestions as to the cause, ranging from the vague physiological statement that changes in the mother's hormones are responsible, to the psychodynamic explanation that the mother is subconsciously trying to reject her baby! It is probably fair to say that the former suggestion seems the more likely but the specific cause is still unknown and that there may be a variety of causes.

This is no comfort to the woman leaning over the kitchen sink every morning and retching. The bland statement by the obstetrician that 'it will soon go away' and 'try and avoid foods that upset you' is no comfort either. Food is furthest from her mind and yet she is acutely aware that she is supposed to be building up those large stores of iron and calcium and protein for the baby.

Unfortunately, there is no certain cure and treatment is very difficult. Drugs which combat nausea are not absolutely safe and it is the usual practice now to avoid giving drugs to a woman during the first 3 to 4 months of her pregnancy if possible, although if the problem is severe the doctor may prescribe one of the safer ones. Many women find that eating *can* help, especially a very light snack (a biscuit or a piece of toast and a cup of tea) eaten before they get out of bed. Serious cases which go on past the third month may have to be treated in hospital. Generally, however, the problem does disappear after the third month and then 'feeding for two' can begin in earnest.

Special appetites during pregnancy often take quite bizarre forms. They are called 'pica', after the Latin word for magpie. A doctor who had taken a special interest in them once showed me a case history card to which was pinned a small square of plastic raincoat. 'She ate the rest!' he said. Another of his patients had felt an uncontrollable urge to eat the stones on the drive, and one night her husband was wakened at 3 a.m. by the police, who had driven past and seen her in her nightdress gobbling up the gravel!

These are rare and extreme examples. Chocolate, or bread and honey, or fresh currant buns, are more usual cravings and more easily obtained and accommodated into the diet of a pregnant woman! The explanation of pica is not known; but it is not serious, and there is no harm indulging in it if the food craved is safe.

14 Feeding athletes

Introduction

Over the past half century human sporting activities have become big business. Footballers are bought and sold like fighting cocks, and sportsmen are paid enormous sums of money for winning a game of golf or tennis. The training schedule for any serious sportsman reads like a countdown for a lunar landing and it is vital to be 'at peak' at the time of the event; if he or she is a professional a misjudgement could cost a great deal of money. The food he eats is part of this training schedule.

The same nutritional principles which apply for good health also apply to good athletic performance. An athlete needs enough carbohydrate, fat, protein, minerals, and vitamins to cover normal needs and extra to cover the increased physical activity and for building bigger muscles. Will additional extra food above these requirements improve his performance? Do big steaks make him stronger? Do extra vitamins help him run faster? Does sugar give him extra energy? It is these questions which are answered in this chapter; they can be summarized under the general headings of extra vitamins, extra protein, and sugar for energy.

Extra vitamins

In a horse-doping case some years ago, a hypodermic syringe discovered in the stable was found to contain traces of vitamin C. At the subsequent enquiry the defence counsel asked whether a shot of vitamin C could be expected to improve the horse's performance. 'Certainly', the expert witness replied, 'if all the horses in the race were suffering from a deficiency of vitamin C and this horse was the only one to receive the vitamin, then it would be at a great advantage over the other competitors.' 'But in the absence of any deficiency?' pressed the counsel. 'In the absence of a deficiency of vitamin C, an injection of the vitamin would not make the slightest improvement to the animal's performance', came the reply.

The same is true for man. An athlete on a mixed diet will be eating adequate amounts of vitamins and there is absolutely no evidence that extra amounts will improve his performance. Athletes do need slightly more vitamins than people leading less vigorous lives, but since they also need (and eat) extra food, this will provide the extra vitamins.

There is a current vogue for extra vitamin E. Recently the members of a football team were given injections of vitamin E in the belief that it would increase their muscle power. Their success rate was unaltered by this treatment. There is absolutely no evidence that extra vitamin E produces faster muscle growth, or more powerful muscles. (In any case, why give injections when vitamin E is active when taken by mouth, as are all vitamins except vitamin B_{12}?)

Extra protein

The vogue for extra animal protein for athletes goes back into ancient history. In Greece, athletes would switch from the largely vegetarian diet of the time to a diet containing lots of meat. Traditionally, warriors have been given extra meat for strength in battle. These changes in the diet of athletes and warriors were quite unnecessary and would have produced no benefit. What has been said about vitamins is true also for protein: enough is enough and extra will not improve performance. Training schedules for some events do result in an increase in the size of muscle, but a normal diet will provide plenty of protein to supply this extra requirement. Nor does the diet need to include meat: a mixed vegetarian diet is perfectly adequate. Some world-class athletes are vegetarians – so, incidentally, are race horses!

Muscle building, which means the incorporation of new protein into muscle, is partly controlled by certain hormones called anabolic steroids. It has sometimes been the practice to administer these hormones, in an effort to produce faster muscle growth. The most potent of these hormones is the male sex hormone, testosterone, and a fringe benefit of such therapy for female athletes is that they might grow a beard! Such hormones have only marginal effects on muscle size in the healthy person who is secreting his or her own anabolic steroids and, since an excess of these hormones has undesirable side-effects, their use has been banned by the World Amateur Athletics Association.

Sugar for energy

Having said that extra protein or extra vitamins will not improve your athletic performance, we come now to extra sugar. The belief that extra sugar gives you energy arises from the knowledge that energy is derived in the body from the breakdown of glucose. The question is, will *extra* sugar give you *extra* energy; in other words, do the supplies ever run out during physical activity?

In order to answer this question, it is necessary to understand how energy is supplied to an exercising muscle. The energy comes from three sources. Firstly, the muscle has its own internal store of glucose built into large molecules called glycogen and stored inside the muscle cells. Secondly, extra glucose can be obtained from the blood. Although the blood contains a total amount of only 5 grams (about a teaspoonful) it is continuously topped up by the liver, which makes glucose from fat and protein, and adds it to the blood. Thirdly, in addition to these two carbohydrate sources, muscle also uses fat, brought by the blood from the fat depots.

When it is functioning efficiently, a muscle uses all three sources of energy. As soon as you start exercising, adrenaline is released, which stimulates the liver and fat depots to release glucose and fat into the blood and thus provide the muscles with energy. The supply of fat is unlimited: a normal man (even a lean one) carries enough fat to provide him with sufficient energy to run 800 kilometres (500 m.)! The carbohydrate stores, however, are not nearly so abundant; in fact they are severely limited. In moderate physical activity the liver can maintain blood sugar for only two to three hours. In very strenuous activity the muscle's own internal store of glycogen is the limiting factor; after only one hour it becomes depleted to a level which significantly reduces performance. Therefore our 'extra sugar for extra energy' has to be directed at replenishing these two carbohydrate stores.

Let's take blood sugar first. A fall in blood sugar has only a minor effect on the muscle, which still has its own glycogen, but the effect on the brain is serious. The brain is almost totally dependent on the blood sugar as a source of energy and if it runs out the symptoms of hypoglycaemia occur: the subject feels dizzy and nauseated, he comes out in a cold sweat, and he may black out. The blood sugar may fall sufficiently to produce these symptoms after only two hours of moderately strenuous exercise. They can be prevented by eating some sugar, which passes from the stomach into the bloodstream in minutes, thus topping up the blood sugar and easing the work-load on the liver.

It is no good taking the sugar before the event because resting muscles will not use it. It will be taken up by the liver and turned into fat and sent on to the fat depots. The sugar must therefore be taken during the event. Nor is it necessary to take glucose; ordinary table sugar is absorbed just as rapidly and is much cheaper. Since dehydration will almost certainly be present owing to increased breathing and to sweating, the sugar should be taken in solution in water. Details are given on page 109.

With very strenuous activity the limiting factor is the glycogen stores in the relevant muscles. These cannot be topped up in a matter of minutes, like the blood sugar. However, in an interesting series of experiments during the last few years it has been shown that the amount of glycogen stored in muscle can be greatly increased by eating a diet rich in carbohydrate. The stores are filled up to even higher levels if they are emptied first by a bout of strenuous exercise. A regime based on these findings is now used by many world-class sportsmen engaged in medium- to long-distance events. For those involved in short events like sprinting or jumping a lot of glycogen is a disadvantage because glycogen is stored with three to five times its own weight of water and therefore filling up the glycogen stores adds weight. This extra weight would be an impediment to the sprinters and the jumpers.

How can all this information be put to practical use for the sportsman?

1. If your event lasts *less than one hour*, there is no advantage to be gained by manipulating the carbohydrate stores.

2. For strenuous events lasting *one hour or longer*, fill up your muscle stores in the following way:
   two days before the event, train heavily; follow this with light training only and a diet rich in carbohydrates (puddings, potatoes, bread and jam) up to the day of the event.
3. For *long-distance* events such as cross-country running or skiing, long-distance cycling or cross-Channel swimming, fill up your glycogen stores as above. In addition, keep your blood sugar up during the event by drinking sugar solution (1–3 teaspoonsful in a glass of water every fifteen minutes).

When to eat

The seaside holidays of my childhood were punctuated by the admonition not to swim after a meal, for fear of getting 'the cramps', and there is a sound reason for this. When a large meal is eaten, blood is diverted to the gut during the process of digestion. This means that if you call on your muscles to do some heavy work at the same time, there will be a competition for the available blood. If the exercise is severe, the muscles may be forced to contract without sufficient oxygen, resulting in painful cramps.

If you are participating in sport for pleasure, it is a good rule not to begin any strenuous physical activity until at least two hours after the end of a meal; also not to make that meal a large or a very fatty one. If you are taking part in competitive sport the last meal should be taken two and a half to three hours before the event, and should contain only foods to which you are accustomed and and which you know from your own experience to be easily digested.

15 Feeding the old, the busy, and the shipwrecked

The old

The commonest nutritional disease in old people in an affluent society is obesity. This problem has been discussed in Chapters 2 and 3.

There are, however, even in an affluent society, old people in lower-income groups who suffer from various forms of under-nutrition: the number in Britain in a survey in 1972 was 3 per cent. Although that is a low percentage it represents 150,000 people, a sizeable group.

There are several reasons why old people tend to be under-nourished. There is a natural reduction in food intake and phys-ical activity with old age, so they tend to eat less. They often live alone, neglecting themselves and not bothering to make sure that their diet has variety. They may be poor and spend very little on food and they may never have learned which cheap foods are also nutritious. With the reduction in food intake and the lack of variety, there is the risk of shortage of certain essential nutrients.

The main deficiencies are vitamins C and D, iron, and protein. For example, old people may not be bothered with fresh fruit and vegetables and they may therefore lack vitamin C; they may not get out into the sunlight much, due to infirmity or depression, and therefore be short of vitamin D; and often they are not able to afford foods such as meat or fish, and do not know how to make up their protein and iron from other sources. These deficiencies can be easily avoided. Extra sunlight is the best way of avoiding vitamin D deficiency. Two hundred and fifty milli-litres (half a pint) of milk a day will give them extra protein and vitamin D. Orange juice, new potatoes, or properly cooked green vegetables will give them vitamin C and also increase their absorption of iron.

If you have an old person in your family, make sure he or she eats these foods and if you know an elderly person living alone find some way of making sure he gets them. Help him to work out how he will include them in his diet; an old person is often loath to change his accustomed way of doing things. Better still, invite him to a meal and give them to him, because loneliness is often a worse problem in old age than the risk of malnutrition.

The busy

There are times when one just seems to be too busy to eat. Mothers looking after small children; business people trying to prepare for an important meeting; actors during the last few days of rehearsal; students before their examinations; brides getting ready for the wedding; people in all sorts of circumstances find it difficult to make time for a proper meal. In addition, a very busy time is often accompanied by fatigue, so that when there is a break in activity there is not the energy to prepare a 'proper meal'. Does it matter? How can one best cope with it?

Firstly, don't bother too much at the busy times about strict dietary principles. The times in question are probably short, no more than a few days or so, and you do not develop dietary deficiencies over a few days even if you eat nothing. Your body stores of fat, vitamins, and protein will tide you over.

What you do need, if you are working hard and rushing around for long periods, is food for energy. Sandwiches are ideal and it does not really matter what the filling is, so choose something you enjoy. Try to have them made with wholemeal bread to give you extra roughage, as you are probably not eating vegetables. Baked beans on toast make a quick meal, as do pilchards or sardines on toast, and all of these have a very high nutritional value and are fairly cheap. Fast food and take-aways are fine for the occasional meal but often use too much salt. If you are really on the run, a 125-gram (5-oz) block of chocolate gives you 3,000 kJ (750 kcal), a quarter of your daily energy requirement. Even better, because it has less sugar, a 100-gram (4-oz) packet of nuts and raisins is as nutritious as a conventional light meal.

For drinking, try milk. It will feed you as well as satisfy your thirst. Alcoholic drinks will provide energy but if you have nothing all day but scotch and soda the side-effects tend to hamper your busy schedule! Tea and coffee are fine once every two hours or so; they contain the stimulant drug caffeine and will 'pick you up', that is they act as a mental stimulant. If you drink them every half hour, however, they may irritate the stomach and have other disturbing effects, like making your heart beat too fast and, if you drink them late at night, they may prevent you getting some much needed sleep.

In short, it is not necessary to sit down to three meals a day, one of them a 'good hot dinner'. Doing so may be pleasant socially and may help your digestion, but has no nutritional advantage over food taken on the run. Remember, however, if your hurried diet goes on for more than a few days make it as *varied* as possible. No one can claim to be in a good nutritional state on a constant diet of fast food, take-aways, or even bread and cheese, if he eats it week in and week out. (Remember also that I have only considered the nutrition side of this question. There are all sorts of other reasons, related to your heart, and even your soul, why life at a leisurely pace may be better for you!)

The shipwrecked

For people awaiting rescue (shipwrecked, aeroplane-crashed, or lost in the mountains) nutrition is not the main problem. If they are not rescued in, say, fourteen days then they will probably not be rescued at all; and in fourteen days even if they have *nothing* to eat they will not starve, let alone suffer from vitamin deficiencies.

Their big nutritional problem is water. A man in a cool climate, and not doing any work, loses an absolute minimum of 1·5 litres (3 pints) of water a day. He cannot prevent this loss. About one-third of it occurs through the lungs as he breathes out moist air; one-third through the skin just by evaporation which occurs without sweating; and the remaining third is lost through the kidneys, excreting a very concentrated urine to get rid of urea and other obligatory waste products.

He can lose only 6 to 8 litres (12 to 16 pints) before he dies from dehydration; therefore at 1·5 litres a day he can survive four to five days if he has no water supply. Any situation which increases this water loss will decrease his survival time – for example, a hot climate, or physical exercise leading to sweating. In extreme circumstances (walking across a desert in a heat wave) a man can die from dehydration in a few hours.

If he is at sea, drinking sea water will do him no good because the concentration of salt it contains is higher than the concentration of salts in his urine. He has to excrete all that salt and he will excrete extra water while doing so. This means that he will dehydrate himself even faster and since delirium is a feature of the final stages of dehydration, this probably accounts for the old sailors' tale that drinking sea water sends you mad. Drinking his own urine will not help either because he will have to excrete all the salts and poisonous wastes again. His only hope is to catch and drink dew or rain water, both of which are free of salt.

Since water is the main problem, survival rations should exclude any foods which increase the need for water. Salt and proteins should be left out, since salt needs water for its excretion, and protein is broken down into urea which also has to be excreted together with water; both will increase the flow of urine. Survival rations should therefore contain only fat and carbohydrate, and since their main function is to boost morale rather than nutrition, they should be as palatable as possible. For most people, that means chocolate!

16 Heart disease

If you are a man over 45 years of age living in a prosperous country, heart disease is more likely to be the eventual cause of your death than anything else. Even for men between 35 and 45, heart disease causes 40 per cent of deaths. These figures are much higher than they were fifty years ago and are still rising, and many people are asking whether they can do anything about it.

Studies to identify the risk factors are not only very difficult to carry out in humans, but very expensive. In 1969 a working party in America calculated that a satisfactory study would cost 213 million dollars; today of course it would cost far more! Consequently the experts have to try and make the best of inadequate studies and conflicting results. However, while the arguments are in progress, it does seem sensible to give some guidance on possible ways of reducing the risk.

Diet is one factor which affects the risk. The question of diet, however, is closely interrelated with other risk factors and for this reason, although this chapter emphasizes the role played by food, the other risk factors are mentioned as well.

What is heart disease?

Heart disease is known to the medical profession as coronary heart disease, because it affects the coronary arteries which carry blood to the heart muscle. With increasing age, fat accumulates in the walls of these vessels, first appearing as fatty streaks in the lining of the artery and later forming disc-shaped raised areas called fatty plaques which bulge out into the vessel and impede the flow of blood.

People with these fatty changes in their arteries may feel pain in the chest when physical exertion begins. This pain arises in the heart, which during physical exertion has to pump with increased force and at an increased rate and so needs more blood for its own muscle. The extra blood cannot be supplied through the narrowed coronary arteries and the pain is due to the insufficient blood supply. The pain is called angina. It can be eased by taking drugs which dilate the coronary vessels. Although the patient may live with angina for many years, his risk of sudden death from a heart attack is high.

Eventually the vessel may close completely, either due to the fatty plaque itself or a clot of blood which forms on it, and a portion of the heart muscle is suddenly deprived of its blood supply. This produces a heart attack. The patient may die or, if he survives, the chance of another attack is high.

This, then, is the pathology of heart disease. It commences at an early age. Soldiers killed in the Vietnam War were studied and some were found to have fatty streaks in their arteries even though they were only 20 years old. People with certain characteristics are much more likely to suffer from the disease. These people are called the 'high-risk' group, and the characteristics which put people in this group are listed in the next section. However, whether you are in the high- or low-risk group you can reduce your own individual risk by taking certain precautions which are described in the last section.

What puts you in the high-risk group?

> Being a man
> Having parents with heart disease
> Being over 45 years old
> Having an obsessive personality
> Suffering from certain diseases

These are the characteristics which increase your chance of having coronary heart disease. Any one of them automatically puts you into the high-risk group. You will notice that it is not a matter of choice; all of them are yours or not by gift, as it were. However, knowing whether or not they apply to you may help you to decide whether to take any of the precautions listed later. Let's have a look at the characteristics in more detail.

Being a man If you are a man, your chances of having coronary heart disease are five times higher than if you are a woman.

Castration helps, but most men would be unwilling to take such extreme measures! However, if you are a woman the sex hormones which are protecting you will turn off at about 45 years of age; after that you gradually enter the high-risk group.

Having parents with heart disease If your parents or grandparents died from a heart attack this increases the risk that you will do the same. Unfortunately, we are not given the opportunity of choosing our parents, any more than they were of choosing us!

Being over 45 years old As stated at the beginning of this chapter, over half the deaths in men over 45 are due to heart disease. These figures were obtained in 1973 and were still rising. The tragic statistic about age, however, is that year by year there is an increase in the number of young men (30–40 years) who die from coronary heart disease.

Having an obsessive personality There is some evidence that your personality may affect the risk. The high-risk personalities have certain characteristics, including obsession with punctuality, worry about meeting deadlines, and great competitive drive. It is the type of personality which matters, and not the type of job; there is no evidence that the executive-type jobs increase the risk. In other words, an obsessive clerk may be more at risk than his easygoing boss.

Suffering from certain diseases There are some diseases which carry an increased risk of heart disease: they include high blood pressure, gout, diabetes, and some abnormalities in fat metabolism which result in high levels of blood fats. If you have any of these, your doctor will already be keeping an eye on you.

What can you do about it?

>Stop smoking
>Be active
>Be thin
>Stop drinking heavily
>Eat less saturated fats and sugar and more fibre

If you are in the high-risk group for coronary heart disease and you wish to reduce the risk, you should follow these suggestions. None of them is guaranteed to be effective, but for all of them the evidence that they reduce the risk is sufficiently strong to make them worthy of your serious effort.

Stop smoking Smoking greatly increases the risk. In fact, lung cancer and bronchitis account for less than half the increased deaths that are seen in smokers; the remainder (over half) are due to coronary heart disease. Smoking twenty cigarettes a day approximately doubles your risk of having a heart attack, so give it up, or cut it down drastically.

Be active It has been shown that bus conductors on double-decker buses have a lower incidence of heart disease than bus drivers, and outdoor postmen a lower incidence than their colleagues in the sorting room. So, if you have a sedentary job, do some exercise every day. The best exercises are those which use large groups of muscles (for example, walking, jogging, bicycling, climbing stairs, or swimming). The important point is: do it hard enough and long enough to get out of breath and make your heart pound, at least once a day. (A friend once said that he did this while making love: would that count? The answer is Yes, and it has the added bonus that it prolongs the life of your chosen partner too!)

Be thin Fat people carry an increased risk (see Chapter 2).

Stop drinking heavily Heavy drinking damages the heart muscle and may also contribute to obesity. Light drinking (one or two a day) won't do you any harm and may even help by making you more relaxed.

Change your diet The more affluent the society, the more frequent the incidence of heart disease. Is this related to changes in our eating habits? People in affluent societies eat more meat, more saturated (animal) fats, more sugar, more alcohol, more tea, more coffee, and, over all, more food. They also eat less fibre.

There is disagreement among medical authorities as to whether any of these is to blame, and the situation is not helped by the energetic propaganda of large business such as the butter, sugar, and margarine industries. For these reasons it is very difficult for the layman to make a sensible decision based on the advice available. He is overwhelmed with conflicting suggestions and he must frequently be tempted to throw his hands in the air and say, 'I'll eat what I like; they'll only think of something else tomorrow!' That's a pity, because if you are in the high-risk group there probably *are* dietary precautions worth taking. The four foods most widely studied are discussed here and they are listed in an order which, most authorities feel, reflects their importance. They are: fats (and cholesterol), carbohydrate, hard water, and salt.

In 1953 the American medical scientist, Ancel Keyes, demonstrated a correlation between the amount of saturated fat eaten by a community and the level of cardiac disease. This finding led to a great deal of research, and finally to the suggestion that eating polyunsaturated fats instead of saturated fats and the reduction of cholesterol in the diet would lower the incidence of heart disease.

To quote some of the findings which seem to support the suggestion that fats and cholesterol play a role in heart disease: the higher the level of cholesterol in the blood, the greater the chance of getting heart disease; the plaques found on the walls of arteries in heart disease contain a lot of cholesterol; eating polyunsaturated fats lowers the blood cholesterol. To put it very simply, what is suggested is that if you eat polyunsaturated fats, your blood cholesterol will fall and this may reduce the formation of fatty plaques on the walls of your arteries.

There are arguments against the theory too. For instance, lowering the cholesterol in the diet does not always reduce the incidence of coronary heart disease. Also, not all studies have demonstrated a fall in the incidence of cardiac disease when a community switched to polyunsaturated fats.

In spite of this controversy, the balance of medical opinion is that a change in the dietary fats is beneficial and high-risk patients should be encouraged to make such a change. In 1976 a joint working party of the Royal College of Physicians of London and the British Cardiac Society published a list of recommendations, and these are reproduced here. If you are in the high-risk group, it is probably wise to follow them.

(a) Eat less meat and fewer egg yolks; eat more poultry and fish. Choose lean meat and remove visible fat from meat. Grill rather than fry.

(b) Use butter sparingly; preferably use a soft margarine high in polyunsaturated fats. In general, avoid cream and the top of the milk.

(c) Use oils rich in polyunsaturated fats for cooking, e.g. corn oil, sunflower oil, safflower oil. Avoid hard margarines or lard. Oils labelled merely 'vegetable oil' may contain a good deal of saturated fat and very little polyunsaturated fat and should be avoided.

(d) Eat more vegetables and fruit of all kinds.

The second food group which may be associated with heart disease is carbohydrate. The British nutritionist, John Yudkin, put forward the theory that sugar is the dietary factor responsible for the increased incidence of heart disease. The evidence is less convincing than it is for fat. However, sugar does have a harmful effect on your teeth, which is indisputable (see Chapter 18). It also consists of empty calories, that is energy associated with no other nutrients, and may therefore contribute to obesity. Since obesity may also be a factor contributing to heart disease, it seems prudent to cut sugar out from the diet if you are in the high-risk group. Eat fewer sweets, puddings, cakes, ice-cream, and biscuits.

It must be stressed that carbohydrates as a whole are not implicated, only sugars. Starchy foods, such as bread and potatoes, are not at all dangerous; indeed, their inclusion in the diet may mean that you eat less fat. Also there is some evidence that dietary fibre (also a carbohydrate) may have a protective effect against heart disease.

The findings about the effect of calcium date back to the observation that people who live in areas where the water is 'hard' have a lower incidence of heart disease than those who live in areas where it is soft. So if you have hard water in your area, don't soften the drinking supply; it may be doing you good. The reasons for this apparent protective effect are so far unknown.

The relationship between salt and heart disease is complex. Firstly, the effect must be separated from the effect of salt on blood pressure. People with high blood pressure are often put on a salt-free diet; this decreases the fluid in their bodies and this in turn lowers the blood pressure. There is, however, a quite separate suggestion that large amounts of salt in the diet will increase the incidence of coronary heart disease. This effect and its implications are discussed in the chapter on minerals (page 84). If you are in the high-risk group, moderate the amount of salt you eat. If you have high blood pressure, your doctor will already have advised you that this is particularly important.

In summary, if you are in the high-risk group, try to modify your diet to reduce saturated fat, sugar, and salt. If you are in the low-risk group, there is probably no need to do so. For either group, no smoking and more exercise are far higher priorities.

17 Food poisoning

In its literal sense food poisoning could mean any poisoning caused by food or drink; a child eating berries from the Deadly Nightshade plant, a Chinese gourmet dying from eating the puffer fish, a man drinking beer contaminated with lead from old-fashioned pipes: all these people have been poisoned by food. However, the term is generally used in a much narrower sense. It means poisoning caused by food or drink which has been contaminated with certain bacteria or viruses.

There is a wide variety of organisms responsible. They produce poisons or toxins and it is these toxins which give rise to the symptoms of food poisoning. The symptoms include headache, vomiting, diarrhoea, abdominal cramps, and a general feeling of weakness.

With the exception of the botulinus organism, the bacteria or viruses live in the bowel. The faeces of an infected person contain living germs and if these faeces are allowed to contaminate food or water, the disease may be passed on to anyone eating or drinking that contaminated material. In poor countries where the sewage and the water supplies are often not well separated (the same river may be used for both), the disease spreads rapidly. The germs may also be present on the skin, so careless handling of food also spreads the disease.

This chapter deals first with gastro-enteritis, which is the general name given to a whole group of diseases caused by eating contaminated food. They are all fairly mild and generally not fatal. They are quite common even in affluent societies but the risks can be reduced and the symptoms treated: I have given some suggestions here. The last part of the chapter is devoted to a brief description of the very serious forms, which include typhoid, cholera, dysentery, and botulism. They are rarely seen in a developed community. They require instant and energetic medical treatment if the patient is to survive.

Gastro-enteritis

When I was a child we used to get a bilious attack, and my uncle used to suffer from Delhi-belly. Other names used are the trots, the runs, or an attack of the gastro! They all refer to gastro-enteritis and the symptoms vary from a vague feeling of discomfort in the gut right through to a decidedly non-vague diarrhoea and vomiting. The disease is an infection; that is, it is due to bacteria or viruses; and one of the ways that it is transmitted from one person to another is by food.

Many kinds of bacteria and viruses produce toxins which cause gastro-enteritis. The exact way in which the toxins work is unknown but the main action seems to be in the gut, where intense irritation occurs. A description of the two major groups, the staphylococci and the salmonellae, will illustrate the different forms of the disease.

Staphylococcal bacteria produce their toxins in the food before it is eaten and the symptoms therefore occur very shortly after eating contaminated food – usually before the next meal. This makes the onset rather dramatic and this feature of the disease has been used by writers of fiction. In one description of an aeroplane flight all the passengers who had eaten fish were struck down with uncontrollable diarrhoea and vomiting. The pilots were also affected, but a brave passenger was able to land the aeroplane to the accompaniment of suitable stirring music. Modern methods of food preparation used by airlines make such happenings unlikely, but dramatic instances do occur in other real-life situations. In one outbreak a women's institute trip to the seaside stopped at a roadside café and ate some contaminated ham sandwiches prepared by a chef who had an infected finger. By the time the excursion reached the seaside the whole bus-load of people was sick. An outbreak affecting the majority of nurses at a hospital was traced to a contaminated shepherd's pie in the staff canteen. Because of the rapid onset of staphylococcal food poisoning, tracing the contaminated food is fairly easy and further cases can usually be prevented.

With salmonella food poisoning the bacteria have to

multiply inside the body before they produce enough toxin to cause symptoms. They multiply in the gut, and it may be one to three days before there are sufficient numbers to produce toxin in large quantities so that quite an interval may elapse before symptoms appear. In order to identify the contaminated food, it is necessary to ask the patient to give a list of all that he has eaten for the previous few days, and this has to be checked against lists from other patients until a food is identified which they have all eaten. People tend to have hazy memories, particularly when they are sick or distressed, and in any case the time interval often means that many more people have eaten food from the same contaminated source. Outbreaks of salmonella food poisoning are therefore more difficult to control.

There are other types of bacteria, and also some viruses, which cause food poisoning: some are like staphylococci and the disease has a rapid onset, others have an incubation period of one to three days like the salmonellae, still others are intermediate in type. The following notes on prevention apply to all of them.

How to prevent gastro-enteritis

The bacteria and viruses which cause food poisoning are present in our environment all the time – in the air, in the soil, everywhere. The reason we don't have food poisoning all the while is because we have built up some immunity to the local organisms. Therefore large numbers are necessary to produce the disease; eating just a few won't harm you.

Knowing the habits of bacteria and the conditions under which they multiply most rapidly will help you prevent heavy contamination of food in your kitchen. Given ideal conditions, one bacterium can divide into two every half hour. This means that in twenty-four hours one bacterium can produce one million million million offspring. Three conditions are needed for this rate of reproduction: food, moisture, and warm temperatures. Bacteria which fall on to warm food (blood heat is the ideal temperature) will find themselves in a perfect environment and will multiply at a very fast rate. For these reasons, warm food should never be left sitting around uncovered. It provides an ideal breeding ground for any bacteria which fall into it and they will start multiplying immediately. You won't be able to see them, smell them, or feel them, and the food may appear to be quite untainted, but it could contain a mass of bacteria ready to play havoc in your gut.

Bacteria are killed by heat. Therefore any cooking process tends to kill them, and the higher the temperature and the longer the cooking the more certain that all the bacteria are killed. Heating at just above boiling point for half an hour kills all bacteria and this is how sterilization is carried out in hospitals. However, boiling for ten minutes will kill most organisms and this is sufficient precaution in the house for food that is to be eaten straight away.

The lower the temperature falls below blood heat, the more slowly the bacteria reproduce. In the refrigerator they are very sluggish, and a deep freeze more or less stops them. (Note: a deep freeze does *not* kill them; see page 126 for hints on defrosting food.) Having this information, it is possible to take precautions which will prevent contamination of food. These precautions are:

> Cook thoroughly
> Cover
> Cool quickly
> Refrigerate

The thorough cooking will kill most of the germs already in the food; covering will prevent more from falling in from the air; cooling and refrigeration will prevent multiplication of any which are still present. Absolute sterility is not needed, but it is important to keep the numbers as low as possible.

In the home, where the volume of food is usually fairly small, following this procedure should eliminate food poisoning. In institutions, however, it is much more difficult. Firstly, the volume of food is greater; a lemon meringue pie half a metre square cools rather slowly! The food cannot be put into the refrigerator until it is cold, because otherwise the steam will condense all over the inside of the refrigerator. To eliminate long periods of warmth, which are ideal for bacterial growth, many institutions are now adding special cooling rooms to their kitchens where large volumes of food are cooled rapidly in forced cold-air draughts.

The second problem in institutions is associated with serving, which may extend over a long period of time. For example, the food prepared for lunch in a factory canteen may be kept warm while three shifts come and go; or in a restaurant food may be partially cooked, kept warm, and then reheated when ordered. The solution to these problems is to avoid pre-cooking as far as possible but, if economics demand it, to keep the cooked food hot enough to prevent bacteria multiplying.

If food does need to be reheated, 'warming through' is not sufficient either to kill any bacteria which may be present, or to destroy their toxins. The food must be thoroughly reheated. The *whole* of the food should be at boiling point (or just below for the gourmet cooks!) for ten to fifteen minutes. Again, large volumes of food are particularly hard to handle; recrisping the potato topping of a large shepherd's pie can leave a seething mass of bacteria in the meat underneath, because large volumes of food heat up slowly and the centre of the pie may only just be warm by the time the top is ready.

Food that is not going to be cooked again (for example, prepared meat like ham) needs special care, whether at home or in a large establishment. It should always be kept cool to reduce multiplication of the bacteria. Also, it should *never* be allowed to touch raw meat. The surfaces of raw meat or raw chicken are frequently contaminated with salmonella bacteria. These will be destroyed when the food is cooked but if they brush off on to meat that is not going to be cooked, they will start to multiply. For this reason, never buy cooked meats from a shop which serves raw and cooked meat at the same counter, and never let raw and cooked meat come into contact on your kitchen table. For example, don't joint a raw chicken and then carve some cooked beef on the same surface, or using the same (unwashed) knife.

I have said very little about conventional cleanliness because on the whole it is rather ineffectual against bacteria. Wiping down the table spreads the bacteria further, and the dish cloth itself is a marvellous breeding ground. Rats, mice, and flies do spread bacteria, but bacterial counts on the kitchen tea towel have shown that the tea towel contains more bacteria than a hundred flies. However, certain rules of personal cleanliness are important while handling food. There are often organisms present in your lower bowel which cause food poisoning, so always wash your hands after going to the toilet. If you have a cut or pimple which is infected, it may contain staphylococci, so keep it well covered. While handling food, don't pick your nose; it is loaded with bacteria. Obviously, these rules for cleanliness apply even more to people who sell food; if you see them ignored, don't go there again.

If you work in a place that sells food or handles large quantities of it, your local health inspector will gladly give you advice on the precautions you should take, and indeed compulsory inspection is often necessary. If you are a person preparing food for the family, the rules for prevention of food poisoning can be summarized as follows:

1. After cooking, cool food as rapidly as possible if storing it.
2. Always cover cooked food.
3. If you reheat food, do so thoroughly.
4. Keep raw meat separate from cooked meat.
5. Practise personal cleanliness while preparing food.

A special note on frozen food

Freezing preserves food but, unlike canning, does not kill all the bacteria; it merely slows them down into a state of suspended animation. This means that frozen food will not keep for ever, the bacteria will eventually spoil it. When food is defrosted, any bacteria present arouse themselves to a state of hyperactivity and at room temperature they multiply rapidly. The danger when defrosting therefore arises if the food is left at room temperature after it has defrosted. This is why it is safer to defrost in the refrigerator; the thawed food will be kept cool and bacteria will multiply only slowly.

If you are faced with sudden guests or (like me) find it impossible to decide at breakfast time what to have for dinner, then you can cook the food straight from the freezer. This is quite safe as long as you cook it for much longer, usually twice as long, otherwise the inside of the food will not get hot enough to kill any bacteria.

This leaves us with the last situation, when the guests are waiting and the food comes out of the freezer in a form in which it cannot be cooked (ten lamb chops three deep in a solid block is the one I always seem to be facing). Defrost it in warm water. The danger is that the outside of the block of food is warm and bacterial multiplication will be rapid, so this method of defrosting means that the food must be cooked *immediately*. Leaving it on the kitchen table for even a couple of hours is dangerous. Also, try to choose cooking methods which give good heat penetration, such as simmering, rather than quick frying or grilling.

You should be safe if you take the following precautions:

When you defrost, try to do so in a refrigerator

If you cook the food frozen, cook for much longer

If you defrost in warm water, cook *immediately and thoroughly*

Frozen chicken and poultry deserves special mention as it poses special problems. It differs from other meats in that it is made up of a combination of thick parts like the legs which thaw slowly, and thin parts like the breast which thaws quickly. Therefore while you are prodding the legs and finding them still rock hard, the bacteria in the breast are already away. Since nearly all poultry is contaminated with salmonellae, there is a big risk of food poisoning if you are careless. Therefore obey the rules even more rigidly for frozen poultry, defrost it in a fridge (twenty-four hours for a chicken, up to three days for a large turkey) or, if you defrost it rapidly, cook it by a casserole method.

Lastly, if your freezer breaks down, can you safely use the food? Any food which is still hard can be safely refrozen for a few weeks. If it has thawed but is still cold, cook it straight away and invite your friends around for a feast. If it is at room temperature, throw it away.

Treatment of gastro-enteritis

The diseases in the gastro-enteritis group are devastating when they strike but not usually dangerous.

Occasionally people do die. The groups in particular danger are the very old and the very young. If the symptoms last for more than twelve hours in an old person or a baby, or twenty-four hours in an adult, or if the patient is prostrated, medical help should be sought immediately.

For mild attacks in otherwise healthy people the best treatment is rest, starvation, lots and lots of fluid, and some salt.

The best fluid is water, boiled if you are not sure of its source. Alcohol and milk should be avoided. If you hate water, try soda water or very dilute cordial. Dip your finger in the salt every hour or so. Don't eat anything; two days' starvation won't hurt you. Rest as much as you can.

Antibiotic treatment is neither necessary nor useful for these mild forms. Most attacks are short and your own antibodies will effectively cure you. As a preventative measure if you are travelling to an area where food poisoning is a serious problem, your doctor may advise Streptotriad (a combination of streptomycin and sulphonamides).

To help stop diarrhoea, kaolin is still probably one of the best and least harmful substances available. Buy it as plain kaolin mixture and take some after every bout of diarrhoea. The recommended dose is too small to be effective so take four times as much (checking first that you have plain kaolin mixture, not kaolin and morphine). If you are travelling, take some kaolin powder with you (easily obtained from the chemist); mix two heaped teaspoonfuls with boiled water and take it after every bout of diarrhoea. This saves having to cope with kaolin mixture leaking all over the clothes in your suitcase! Lomotil tablets are effective in preventing diarrhoea. These act by stopping movement in the gut; they were given to astronauts to stop their bowel movements (for obvious reasons) on short space flights. However, the tablets contain atropine, which is quite a dangerous drug, and are therefore available only on prescription; they have undesirable side-effects if taken too often. To prevent vomiting, travel sickness tablets are sometimes effective. The antihistamine types are the safest; the other kind of travel sickness pill contains atropine-like drugs and taking too many is dangerous. The chemist will tell you which is which. Never take Lomotil at the same time as these atropine-type tablets, or you are doubling the atropine dose.

Remember that you get food poisoning when travelling because you have no protective antibodies against the local resident bacteria. This explains why the Indian guide can drink the water of the Ganges but you can't; and why your host in New York can eat steak tartare but you must not. While in transit, eat only thoroughly cooked food if possible. Avoid fruit unless peeled, milk and water unless boiled, sliced pre-cooked meat, and

peeled, milk and water unless boiled, sliced pre-cooked meat, and
any dishes which you suspect may have been sitting around warm
for some time, like the egg custard on the dessert trolley or the
salmon mayonnaise.

The serious forms

With these forms of food poisoning, there is a very high risk of the
patient dying. They include cholera, when the patient can die in
twenty-four hours from fluid loss due to copious diarrhoea;
typhoid, in which some of the bacteria move out of the gut into
the blood, causing a general infection all over the body; and
dysentery, in which the bacteria live mainly in the large bowel.

In communities with poor standards of hygiene, these
serious diseases are always present to some degree and they may
suddenly flare up into an epidemic. With the limited medical
resources available, many thousands of people may die, including
a high proportion of children. In developed communities, the
diseases are rare owing to strict control of sewage disposal,
sterilization of drinking water, and compulsory inspection of
premises distributing food. Suspected cases can be isolated and
given intensive medical treatment and the patient often recovers.

The most serious (although very rare) disease caused by
bacterial contamination is botulinus poisoning. This is caused by
the botulinus organism, which produces one of the most powerful
toxins known. The toxin is a nerve poison. Nerves normally
transmit their messages to muscles by releasing a chemical,
acetylcholine, on to the surface of the muscle. The effect of
botulinus toxin is to prevent the release of acetylcholine so that
all the muscles of the body are paralysed. The patient cannot even
breathe, because the muscles of respiration are paralysed. In some
cases patients can be kept alive on artificial respirators until the
effects of the poison wear off, but the disease is often fatal.
Symptoms do not develop for several days, so the contaminated
food is often difficult to trace.

Outbreaks of botulism have been associated with home-
canned or -bottled fruit and vegetables, indicating that during
preparation the heating process has not been sufficient to kill all
the bacteria; or that the container has not been sealed properly
and bacteria have entered after the food has been processed.

Commercial canning processes are much more rigidly controlled, although very rarely accidents do happen; an outbreak of botulism in Britain in 1978 was due to a tin of salmon. One of the cans had a tiny (invisible) hole in its seam and during the canning process the heated cans were cooled in cold running water. Some water was sucked into the can and a botulinus bacterium probably entered with the water. One organism would have been sufficient; it would have multiplied into many inside the can. Other sources are pre-cooked meats, for example ham or salami-type sausages. These should never be eaten if there is any evidence of spoilage either in appearance or smell. Cases of botulism have, however, occurred from eating food which appeared perfectly sound.

There is very little you can do personally to guard against these serious forms of food poisoning. You have to rely on government bodies to protect you. For example, to protect ourselves from such epidemics in overcrowded urban communities, one of the prices we pay is called the water rates! In countries which are underdeveloped, overcrowding soon leads to outbreaks of serious food poisoning and, in affluent communities, events such as floods or fires which damage sewage and water systems are accompanied by a similar risk.

18 Tooth decay

Although tooth decay occurred in ancient times, it did so only rarely, as the teeth dug up from ancient graveyards testify. Now it has reached astonishing proportions. In 1979 in Britain, 17,000 15-year-olds had false teeth and 3 out of 10 people over 16 had lost all their teeth. In Australian country towns, a 'full set of uppers and lowers' was frequently a present for an eighteenth birthday: 'Have all your teeth out, sonny, they'll only cause you trouble!' And sonny did; he had suffered so much toothache as a child that he was easy to convince!

There are many advantages in the prevention of tooth decay. These include financial savings: a great deal of the dentist's time is spent on treating tooth decay and not having to do it would reduce health bills substantially. There are also nutritional advantages, although these are not related to chewing. Food swallowed whole is adequately broken down by digestive juices; your mother's admonition to chew each mouthful a hundred times may have saved you from indigestion but was not essential from the nutritional point of view. However, people with no teeth, or false teeth, tend to avoid certain foods such as apples and meat and so reduce the variety in their diets, and a reduction in variety always raises the danger of dietary deficiencies.

The reason dental disease appears in a book on food is that it is caused directly by one constituent of the diet (sugar) and made worse by a deficiency of another (fluoride). Correction of these nutritional faults would eradicate the disease.

Sugar

Eating sugar is the primary cause of dental decay. In his book *Pure, White and Deadly* Yudkin quotes a German visitor to the court of Queen Elizabeth I in 1598 who, on his return home, described the Queen's black teeth and commented that 'this was a defect the English seem subject to from their too great use of sugar'. Since that comment, the connection between sugar and dental decay has been established over and over again. Eskimos living on diets with no sugar suffered very little dental decay until 'civilization' arrived; their consumption of sugar then increased dramatically and so did their rate of tooth decay. Australian aborigines have been similarly affected and there are many other examples.

The sugar causes teeth to decay because it is broken down by bacteria in the mouth to form acid, which attacks the enamel. Every tooth is coated with enamel, which is very tough, but not tough enough to resist the action of acid. Once the enamel is broached the inside softer part of the tooth is attacked and a cavity appears. Also the bacteria form a very firm coating on the teeth called plaque, which cuts the teeth off from the normal cleansing action of saliva.

As discussed in the chapter on carbohydrates, it is not easy to exclude sugar if you live in modern Western society. Perhaps the best to be hoped for is a reduction in the amount of sugar eaten, together with an avoidance of the more dangerous forms. The dangerous forms are the sticky ones, because they adhere to the teeth for longer periods, giving the bacteria in the plaque a chance to break the sugar down into acid. Such foods as toffees, biscuits, dried fruits, and cakes are the really bad culprits, particularly if they are eaten between meals so that the debris stays in the mouth for a long time. Boiled sweets are not so bad as the sugar is in solution and is washed off the teeth by the saliva, and sugary foods taken with meals are also less harmful as the teeth are usually cleaned after a meal. If you can avoid toffees, biscuits, dried fruits, and cakes between meals, you will do a lot to prevent tooth decay. Soft drinks are also a hidden trap; they nearly all contain a lot of sugar and on a hot day the teeth may be bathed in a constant stream of sugar solution. The low-calorie ones avoid this problem, but too much of these will lead to an undesirably high intake of artificial sweeteners. Better still, suggest to the children that water will quench their thirst!

Fluoride

In an ideal world, recognition of sugar as the cause of tooth decay would inevitably lead to a cure. We would all stop eating sugar. However, decades of warning by the dental profession have gone unheeded, mainly because they spend less on advertising than the confectionery firms do, but also because people love sugar! Therefore we have to look at methods of preventing tooth decay.

Fluoride is an element closely related to calcium; if it is present in the food, it becomes built into tooth enamel. Tooth enamel containing fluoride is much more resistant to attack by acid. Therefore if fluoride is taken it makes teeth stronger and dental decay is reduced.

People who live in areas where the water contains fluoride have less tooth decay than those whose water contains no fluoride. This fact has been established over and over again. It has been established in natural situations: two villages on each side of a mountain had different water supplies, and the teeth of the children from the fluoride village showed a much lower incidence of decay than did those from the non-fluoride village. It has also been established in situations in which fluoride is added to the water by the local authorities: the incidence of dental decay decreases dramatically. There is a great deal of evidence of this nature, and very few people now argue about the effectiveness of fluoride in decreasing tooth decay.

What people do argue about, and with single-minded fervour, is the right of local authorities to add fluoride to the water supply when the natural fluoride content is low. Two arguments are used to support the objection.

Firstly, it is argued that once a water supply is fluoridated there is no alternative supply and therefore fluoridation threatens the basic human right of freedom of choice. These claims must be considered carefully. Throughout history many many wrongs have been done to people 'in their own interests'. The rationale for the tortures of the Inquisition was the benefit of the miscreant, who had no freedom of choice! However, in a civilized society a balance has to be struck between individual liberty and the common good; it is one of the responsibilities of the law to protect this balance. Fluoridation battles have to be fought in courts of law; usually the balance has been in favour of fluoridation.

The second argument used is that fluoride is harmful. Most of the scientific evidence suggests just the opposite: populations drinking water with *very high* amounts of fluoride (10 parts per million) have shown no difference from populations drinking low fluoride *except* that their teeth were better! Every known harmful effect is searched for in tests of this kind. People on the very high fluoride showed no increase in incidence of cancer, or heart disease, they lived for the same length of time, their birth rates were normal, no deformities in babies were noted, and everything else which might be tested was normal. The *only* undesirable effect was an occasional black mottling of the teeth, but this does not occur at the recommended level of fluoridation, which is one part per million.

On balance, it seems to me that water supplies in low fluoride areas should have extra fluoride added. This is not always done; you can ring your local authority and ask them for the fluoride level in your water. If it is below one part per million, and if you want to decrease tooth decay, give fluoride tablets to your children until they are 12 years of age. If you are giving them to babies, the tablets will have to be dissolved in the milk, but give them to older children to chew between meals as soon as they are able, as milk tends to prevent the absorption of fluoride. The tablets are quite tasteless.

Does cleaning your teeth do any good?

There are two benefits derived from cleaning your teeth (apart, that is, from the social benefit of making you nicer to be near!).

The first benefit is the removal of the debris in your mouth after eating, thus preventing sugary particles from lying around and being broken down by bacteria. Bacteria swing into action in the mouth as soon as the sugar arrives, so to be effective teeth cleaning should take place immediately after eating. If it is done properly, it will help prevent tooth decay. It is, however, important to do it properly: your dentist will tell you how—but briefly, round and round with a soft toothbrush is the correct method.

The second benefit is the prevention of periodontal disease, a disease of the gums. This disease is associated with formation of calculus, a deposit containing calcium which forms along the teeth margins in the gums. In communities where abrasive and tough matter is chewed, calculus does not develop and disease of the gums is rare. Careful cleaning of the teeth prevents calculus formation and protects against periodontal disease. Again, ask your dentist to demonstrate the correct method.

Toothpaste is not very effective as a cleaning agent, its main function being to make the mouth and toothbrush smell nice. In the 1950s chlorophyll was added and we all cleaned our teeth with green paste containing 'nature's own deodorant'—pretty, but useless. Now we are given fluoride toothpastes. These do have a beneficial effect, since it has been shown that local application of fluoride to the teeth reduces tooth decay. So choose a toothpaste which appeals to you because it tastes and smells nice, and make sure it contains fluoride.

Chewing raw carrots or apples has been often suggested as a method of clearing the teeth of sugary debris. In an experiment to test whether they worked, some valiant volunteers chewed either raw apple or carrot for an hour after every meal. They developed very strong jaw muscles, but they also developed as much plaque on their teeth as did the subjects who chewed no apples. In fact, peanuts and cheese were found to be more effective; they stimulated the flow of saliva but were not sugary or acid, as apples are. A recent editorial on the subject in the *British Medical Journal* ended with the following statement: 'So, while apples must be demoted from their position of eminence as foods "good for teeth", other foods, among them peanuts and cheese, which are harmless to the teeth and help to combat the effects of potentially harmful foods might be recommended both as between-meal snacks and as the last item of the diet at mealtimes' (April 1977).

19 Nutrition, cancer, and old age

This chapter presents the growing evidence that both longevity and the incidence of cancer can be altered by the food you eat. The evidence so far is largely circumstantial, but the indications are intriguing and certainly sufficiently strong to justify some modifications in the modern Western diet.

Firstly, longevity is discussed: is there a possibility of living longer if the amount of food is restricted? Secondly, cancer: does anything in food cause cancer; can diet protect you from cancer; and what is the association between obesity and cancer? Lastly, since we all clutch at straws when it comes to cancer and old age, the chapter ends with a caution; a warning against claims that any change in your diet will keep you young for ever, or melt a tumour away.

Longevity

Although the age at which you die is determined largely by the species to which you belong and by heredity, it is affected to some extent by factors which are under your own control. For those living in a modern Western society, whether you smoke is probably the most important of these factors; they also include excessive alcohol consumption, which shortens life, daily exercise, which may lengthen life, and now there is growing evidence that longevity may be affected by the food you eat.

Experiments suggest that it is how much rather than what you eat which is important. The first evidence came in 1935 from an experiment on rats. Animals fed on the standard laboratory diet and allowed to eat as much as they wanted for the whole of their lives had an average life span of 656 days. Similar rats were restricted in the first year of their lives to a quantity of food that allowed them to gain no weight at all. Many died, this level of restriction being very severe, but the survivors lived for an average of 835 days, an increase in longevity of 20 per cent.

This experiment has been repeated many times with variations. Scientists have used different animals (mice, hamsters), and different periods of restriction (first year of life, second year of life, alternating weeks throughout life); the over-all results are the same. Animals subjected to any restriction in the quantity of food allowed will live longer than animals with free access to food throughout life.

Are these results applicable to man? Nobody knows. Small animals such as rats and mice have a high metabolic rate and may be more susceptible to the influences of diet and growth rate. Larger animals have longer life spans and experiments would take half a century instead of a couple of years and have therefore not been done. Experiments on man, apart from being unethical, would produce no results for a hundred years! However, it is known that obesity in man is associated with a decrease in the life span. This fact, taken together with the animal experiments described, suggests that in our society being frugal rather than over-indulgent with food will increase the chance of longevity.

Does anything in food cause cancer?

For many years it was believed that cancer was an inevitable accompaniment of ageing and that little could be done to prevent it. This view has now been challenged by many people. Sir Richard Doll, one of the leading researchers in Britain in this field, has pointed out that most, if not all, cancers are caused by agents in the environment and could be prevented by the removal of these agents. He places the identification of these environmental hazards as one of the highest priorities in cancer research, with the possibility of a dramatic reduction in the incidence of cancer if the research proves successful.

Some of the environmental hazards are well known. They include smoking, atomic radiation, and industrial agents such as asbestos and chemicals used in the dyeing trade. Other hazards are not yet recognized and every advance in technology is accompanied by risk. Some of this risk is associated with food.

Hazards in food may occur naturally: a fungus which grows on peanuts produces the poison aflatoxin which causes liver cancer. Others are artificially introduced: certain food additives have been shown to produce cancer in experimental animals when administered in very high doses: the artificial sweetener cyclamate, and the preservative nitrite, are discussed in Chapter 20. In the battle to identify and prohibit the hazards which may produce cancer, the composition of food is therefore an important consideration. Rigid controls have been introduced but mistakes may still occur. What can you do to ensure that you and your family are protected?

The list of additives in current use is long and constantly changing and the evidence against any particular additive is difficult to assess unless you are an expert. However, commercially processed foods are the main source of additives and while their moderate use poses little danger, obviously any risk is reduced if you do not allow these foods to form the major part of your diet. To give one example: one or two artificially flavoured drinks a day may be safe, but on a very hot day a child may drink a dozen such drinks and this may be an unacceptably high intake of artificial additives.

Can diet protect you from cancer?

Just as some food constituents may cause cancer, others may protect you against the disease. Two such constituents currently arousing interest are vitamin A and dietary fibre.

As early as 1926 it was recorded that rats on a diet deficient in vitamin A developed cancers of the stomach. In 1976 in a similar experiment rats were maintained on a diet low in vitamin A; these rats developed four times as many experimental tumours as a similar group kept on a diet containing adequate vitamin A. These experiments and many others with similar results suggest that adequate vitamin A in the diet protects against the *development* of cancer in rats. In addition, it has been shown that vitamin A painted on to skin tumours in mice sometimes caused a reduction in the size of the tumour. It was, however, totally ineffective against other types of tumours.

What do these experiments tell us about cancer in man? The animal experiments all use tumours induced artificially by chemical agents: obviously similar experiments cannot be carried out in man. However, a study carried out by Japanese scientists is pertinent. Over a period of ten years (and still continuing) records of dietary habits and other activities were collected from more than a quarter of a million adults over 40 years of age and correlated with their diseases and causes of death. This study suggests that the incidence of several types of cancer is lower in those people who included in their daily diet a serving of green-yellow vegetables or some milk. Green-yellow vegetables are those containing a lot of the vitamin A precursor carotene (carrots, spinach, green peppers, pumpkin, kale, green cabbage, Brussels sprouts); milk of course is a rich source of vitamin A. The study showed that even the high risk of lung cancer in smokers was reduced by a regular intake of these foods.

There is therefore some evidence that adequate vitamin A will protect against the development of some forms of cancer in man. However, repeated trials to demonstrate an effect of vitamin A once the disease is established have not shown any effect and have had to be abandoned because too much vitamin A is toxic. Vigorous research is now being directed towards finding non-toxic analogues of vitamin A which will reduce tumour size.

On a mixed diet in an affluent society, your diet almost certainly contains adequate vitamin A; if you want to be especially sure, dairy products and green-yellow vegetables are the best sources and the vegetables are better as they contain no animal fat. Taking excess vitamin A has no established effects on cancer and will poison you. Meanwhile, the results of further research are obviously awaited with great interest.

Dietary fibre is the second food constituent which may provide protection against cancer, specifically cancer of the colon. The evidence is based on the observation of Denis Burkitt, who spent much of his life working in Africa. He noted that cancer of the colon was far less prevalent in his rural African patients than it was in Europeans and he speculated that this might be due to the protective effect of the high dietary fibre content of the African diet. Many observations on the relationship between dietary fibre and cancer of the colon in different societies have been made since and most of them support Burkitt's suggestion.

There are several theories as to how fibre acts as a protection against cancer of the colon. This part of the bowel is the home of a large population of harmless bacteria which alter the contents as they pass through it. Many products are formed in the process and some of them are carcinogens (substances which produce cancer). Especially prominent as a source of carcinogens are the bile salts, which are secreted in the bile if there is any fat in the diet. The Western diet, with its high fat content, stimulates a high secretion of bile salts; thus the level of carcinogens in the bowel of Western man is likely to be high. Fibre may help this situation in several ways: by diluting the bowel contents and thus diluting any carcinogens present; by speeding up bowel emptying and thus allowing less time for carcinogens to act on the lining of the bowel; by changing the bacterial population to one which produces less carcinogens; or by binding bile salts so that they are not broken down.

It is only fair to say that, while all these modes of action are theoretically possible, none has been proved by experiment. However, fibre does carry other nutritional advantages (see Chapter 5). The modern Western diet is low in dietary fibre and high in animal fat and it would certainly improve health if the fibre content were increased by eating more wholegrain cereal, fruit, and vegetables. Any possible protective action against cancer would be an added advantage.

Obesity and cancer

The most important effect of obesity on the incidence of cancer is related to breast cancer. This is the most common cancer in women and there are many factors which increase its incidence, including the early onset of menstruation and a family history of the disease. Of interest here is the finding that the disease occurs more frequently in women who are obese.

The reason for this may be related to oestrogens (female sex hormones). Oestrogens are necessary for the development of breast cancer. These hormones are secreted by the ovaries and this source disappears after the menopause. However, adrenal hormones can be converted into oestrogens in the fat tissue, and it has been suggested that the excess fat tissue in an obese woman increases the amounts of oestrogens formed and the risk of breast cancer is therefore raised.

Conclusions

In this chapter, all the evidence about the effect of diet on old age and cancer is circumstantial. Much of it is obtained from animal studies and may not be applicable to man. Much of it is epidemiological, that is related to average figures for specific groups of people: for those belonging to the low-risk group the risk is reduced but not removed. For these reasons, assumptions from the evidence should not be exaggerated. There is no elixir of youth. Carrots do not cure cancer, neither does any other food, whereas radiation therapy, surgery, and drugs do. Whatever you decide to do about your diet, the best hope for cancer is *early diagnosis* followed by conventional treatment, so if you think you have the disease, see a doctor immediately.

However, the measures which reduce the risks are simple to follow; they are also harmless or even beneficial. Thus food restriction in a Western society may not guarantee a longer life, but it confers many other advantages which make it worth while. Similarly, eating a diet with adequate vitamin A or extra dietary fibre will not guarantee that you won't have cancer, but it will improve your health in many other ways, so the chance that it may protect you against cancer is an added bonus!

20 Processed food and food additives

Say 'processed food' to most people – which foods spring into their minds? Long-life milk, TV dinners, soup in a cup, instant puddings, tinned peas: all of these would be thought of as processed food, and indeed they are. But so is farmhouse butter, a wedge of Cheddar cheese, and a slice of homemade wholemeal bread. Processed food is any food which is prepared; that is, not eaten raw off an animal or out of the ground. Processed foods have existed ever since man cooked his first piece of meat over a fire.

Man is the only animal to treat food in any way before he eats it. He did so in the first case probably because he preferred the taste of cooked food to raw food. He later learned that by processing food he could preserve it and so extend the season of plenty. Nowadays he eats even more processed food, partly for convenience but mainly because the giant food-processing firms combine with the advertising industry to persuade him to do so. There is now a wide variety of processed foods available in developed countries, and more and more of what we eat comes into this category.

This trend has led many people to wonder whether processed foods are bad for you. Food is considered to be 'not the same as it used to be': modern bread has the consistency of cotton wool, chickens are tasteless, eggs don't have yellow yolks, and it even seems impossible to make a decent pot of tea. It all adds up to a general uneasiness that the food we are eating is not doing us as much good as it used to.

This chapter examines the nutritional value of processed food. Were we better off in Grandma's day? What about tinned and frozen foods? Are food additives dangerous? And lastly, what are the effects in terms of world resources; is food processing a wise economy or a wicked waste?

Were we better off in Grandma's day?

When you hear people say that food is not like it used to be, they are usually referring to the flavour. The tastes we enjoyed in childhood are often associated with a happy and secure time of our lives, and when we are grown up we embark on a fruitless search to regain ill-remembered and highly subjective sensations.

In some cases, flavours *have* changed. Farming methods have altered; for example, the flavour of bread changes as new pest-resistant strains of wheat are introduced and the flavour of chicken meat is altered by the food the chickens are given. However, although flavours have changed, there is absolutely no evidence that either modern farming methods or modern food technology produces food which is less nutritious. For example, the composition of eggs from battery hens and free-range hens has been analysed and no difference found in their respective nutritional values. The free-range eggs had browner shells and yellower yolks, but we don't eat the shells and the yellow pigment in the yolk (xanthophyll) has no nutritional value. To take another example, the modern hamburger or sausage may well have only a nodding acquaintance with real meat, but the soy bean protein it contains is just as good for you; it has the same amino acids in approximately the same proportions.

In affluent countries we are, in fact, better off than we were in Grandma's day. In affluent societies nutritional diseases are seen only rarely. There are several other measurable signs that nutrition has improved: we are taller, children reach puberty earlier, and fewer small babies are born. One of the reasons for the improvement is that there is more money available today to buy food. In addition, many essential food factors are added to cheap staple foods: thus margarine has vitamins A and D added to it, flour is fortified with calcium, and water is fluoridated. Many of these changes were brought about during the Second World War, when the general nutritional status in some countries, for example Britain, was better than ever before in spite of severe rationing.

However, there is another change in affluent countries which is not beneficial. Some foods which may be harmful are more readily available. For example, meat was quite a luxury fifty years ago; many households bought only one joint a week and the whole of Sunday morning was devoted to roasting 'the joint', with much discussion of its quality while it was being eaten. Then, after the Second World War, standard breeding, slaughtering, and packaging processes led to the appearance of convenient standard joints in see-through packages in the supermarkets, and this ready availability, coupled with greater prosperity, led to an increase in the consumption of meat. Another change of this kind is the increased consumption of sugar. Sugar and all its products were luxuries a hundred years ago; now every corner shop displays a tempting variety of different confectionery in the form of sweets and cakes and biscuits, all within range of our pockets.

This ready availability of various processed foods has contributed to problems such as obesity, tooth decay, and heart disease: modern man's diseases in an affluent, supermarket society. In these respects, we may have been better off in Grandma's day!

Do processed foods contain any goodness?

Processed foods come in a very wide variety of fancy packages, but basically one of two methods has been used in their preparation: either heat, or cold. Heat is used in cooking, drying, and canning; cold is used for storage in frozen and refrigerated foods. Therefore the question we are really asking is: does heat or cold destroy (or reduce) the nutritional value of the fats, carbohydrates, proteins, vitamins, and minerals present in food?

Fats are hardly changed at all by heat. At very high temperatures, such as those used in deep frying, small quantities of the fats polymerize; that is, the molecules join together to form large molecules. These large molecules may alter the flavour of the fat and they have been shown to be toxic to laboratory animals, although there is no evidence that they harm humans. However, it may be prudent not to eat fried food every day and, when deep frying, not to let the temperature of the fat get too high or use the fat too many times.

Proteins are often changed in appearance by heat. Eggs and meat are obvious examples: egg white changes from a liquid into a white solid, meat changes colour from red to brown owing to changes in the pigment of the muscle protein. These changes, however, do not alter the nutritional value of the protein except in very extreme cases, for example the protein on the outside of roasted meat may be cooked to a hardness which makes it impenetrable to digestive juices; conversely, the gelatine in the Chinese dish of shark's-fin soup is unavailable to digestion until it is made soluble by a long period of slow cooking. Canning does not use such extremes and the nutritive value of tinned protein is the same as that of fresh protein.

Carbohydrates are made more available by heat, because in the natural state they are enclosed inside the impervious plant cell walls and these are disrupted by cooking. Raw whole rice, for example, would pass through the intestine largely unchanged, but boiled rice is easily digested. After toasting, carbohydrate is even more quickly digested because some of the starches are broken down into smaller molecules on the outside browned surface. Heating can therefore increase the nutritional value of carbohydrate by increasing the amount available.

Minerals in food are unaffected at any temperature used in cooking. However, their concentration may be decreased by excessive washing or boiling. Other processes may increase the mineral content; thus hard water raises the calcium content of food. Cooking vessels may add minerals too; iron pots used by the Bantu in Africa add iron to the food during cooking and excess iron is found in the tissues of people of this tribe. Copper pots will add copper to food and since excess copper is poisonous, these pots are often coated with tin on the inside. Canned food is packed in cans made of steel, which would add iron to the food, so the inside of the can is coated with tin. Food left in an opened can may absorb a little iron from the cut surfaces, but the amount picked up by the food in this way does no harm at all. (It may change the taste slightly. After the can is opened it is best to decant the food into a dish if you want to keep its taste unchanged.)

This leaves the vitamins, and these are the only constituents of food which are destroyed by heat. The two which are lost to a significant extent are vitamin B_1 and vitamin C (see page 77). Vitamin B_1 is so widely distributed that its partial loss does not pose a nutritional hazard. This is not true for vitamin C. If you live mainly on tinned food, you should take a supplement of vitamin C.

Dehydration is another way of processing food using heat

and again the only component to suffer is vitamin C. Thus dried milk or dried eggs are just as nutritious as fresh milk or fresh eggs, which contain no vitamin C anyway. (This is not to say they taste the same; many people will have eaten dried eggs and will know that they taste *nothing* like real eggs! But they are just as nutritious.) Dried fruit and vegetables lose most of their vitamin C, so sultanas, dates, dried apricots, and all the other delicious dried fruits have none at all. Freeze drying (instant coffee, some vegetables) uses less heat, and may preserve vitamin C during the actual processing; however, the product is often kept on the shelf for a long time and the content of vitamin may be low at the time of eating.

The other major food-processing method used is cold. The food is usually frozen while it is very fresh and is unchanged nutritionally by the process. In fact, since vitamin C is more stable at very low temperatures, the vitamin C content is maintained better than it is in fresh food, which may be days or even weeks travelling from field to kitchen. The only danger with frozen food is related to bacterial contamination when it is thawed; the avoidance of this is described in Chapter 17.

Does all this mean that nothing is wrong with processed food?

Having said that, apart from vitamin C, processed food does not lose its nutritive value, one is still left with an uneasy feeling: surely simple, natural food must be better?

In a way, this doubt is justified; there are disadvantages of processed food. However, these are related not to loss of nutritional value but to the addition of various ingredients. You often do not know exactly what is in processed foods. There are labelling laws, but the information appears in small print while the picture on the label is large and tempting and does not show the additives.

The ingredient which is most commonly added is sugar. This might be expected in products like canned fruit and soft drinks although the amounts might surprise you. One-quarter of the weight of canned fruit may be sugar; a can of soft drink such as Coca Cola contains up to a tablespoonful per glass, and even 'adult' soft drinks like tonic water and bitter lemon have one to two teaspoonsful of sugar in a normal serving. However, sugar also lurks in unexpected places. A small glass of tomato juice has a heaped teaspoonful; nearly all muesli-type cereals have a lot of added sugar; and it is there adding cheap bulk to your children's baked beans and peanut butter. Therefore, when you eat processed food, even if you avoid the obviously sweet ones, you are increasing your consumption of sugar. The dangers of this are discussed in Chapter 5.

Chemical additives

The other common additives to processed food are various chemicals, which are added to preserve food, to colour it, or to add to its flavour.

For centuries chemicals have been added to food to preserve it. Acetic acid (vinegar) has been used to preserve onions and many other vegetables; saltpetre (potassium nitrate) has been used in the curing of bacon; and sodium chloride (salt) has been used to store herrings. Not many of us think of pickled onions, bacon, or salted herrings as dangerous. Tradition and time have given them respectability, and indeed these are not bad criteria. In more recent times a large number of new food additives have been introduced without tradition and time to prove their safety but with the benefit of extensive laboratory tests for their toxicity.

Many people have become very worried about the increasing use of food additives and they wonder if there are sufficient constraints on their use. It would take too much space to list the arguments for and against all the chemicals now used, and anyway the list would quickly be out of date. The problems are well illustrated by three of the better known controversies: cyclamates, nitrates, and fluoride.

Cyclamates are artificial sweeteners discovered in the 1940s. At that time, another artificial sweetener, saccharin, was being used. Saccharin is three hundred times sweeter than sugar but it leaves a bitter after-taste; cyclamate is only thirty times sweeter than sugar but has far less after-taste. Tests on rats showed that quantities of cyclamate far higher than humans were likely to eat produced only one side-effect: a slight laxative action. Cyclamate therefore widely replaced saccharin as an artificial sweetener because it lacked the bitter after-taste. Then several years later it was discovered that some people convert cyclamate to cyclohexylamine in their bodies, and cyclohexylamine is more toxic than cyclamate. However, the use of cyclamate was still allowed. Later still, it was found that cyclamate itself was toxic in the guinea pig, producing liver damage at doses only a few times greater than the maximum recommended intake for man. Still cyclamate was not banned. Then quite suddenly it *was* banned, on the far less damaging evidence that enormous doses of cyclamate *in combination with saccharin* were found to produce occasional breast cancer in rats.

Nitrates, one of the old and established food additives, have been used for years to preserve meat. In the early part of this decade it was discovered that nitrates can be changed into compounds called nitrosamines. This change occurs by bacterial action either in the food itself or in the stomach of the person eating the food. Nitrosamines were shown to cause cancer of the liver in rats, even when given in very small doses. Nitrates are not banned, they are still used in the preservation of meat, especially bacon.

Finally, fluoride. The fluoride story is told in detail in the chapter on dental decay. Briefly, fluoride cannot be shown to be harmful even when used in large doses. The reports that it causes a variety of diseases have all failed to be confirmed on careful investigation, and the World Health Organisation has issued a statement suggesting that the use of fluoride poses no dangers. In spite of this, many local authorities still ban the addition of fluoride to the water.

So there we have three examples: cyclamate, its use allowed for years and then banned in a panic on poor and irrelevant evidence; nitrates, not banned although there is evidence that they are dangerous; fluoride, proved both safe and beneficial and its use still banned by some authorities. There seems to be no logic in these actions. How well is the consumer protected?

As with many contentious areas in the nutrition field, it is difficult to summarize, or to make absolute statements. Any new food additive is subject to stringent tests to prove its safety before its use is allowed. None of the additives will do harm in small doses and it is probable that most are safe at levels far higher than those consumed by most people. However, the price of safety, as with liberty, is eternal vigilance, and it is the function of pressure groups to be both vigilant and vociferous, thereby preventing an insidious overuse of food additives.

To avoid danger, be cautious with manufactured processed foods of unknown composition. Use them as convenience foods or for special occasions, but do not let any single product form your staple diet. That way you can be safe without being needlessly overcautious.

Wise economy? Or wicked waste?

Food processing started as an economic measure. The glut of summer milk was turned into cheese to be eaten during the winter months. Smoked cod or pickled mussels are preserved forms of two fish which have a short winter season. The pig, often the only meat available to a poor family, could be spread over many months by turning some of its meat into bacon. In all these ways, a glut of food was husbanded so that it was spread over leaner times. Processed food was a wise economy, and used in this way it still is.

Gradually, however, food processing has moved out of the home and into the factory. This has brought many benefits to the housewife, who can now serve lamb and green peas all the year round, salmon whenever she wants to (out of the freezer or a tin), and fresh cream teas to unexpected visitors because she has some long-life cream in the fridge. It has also brought benefits to the busy, who can finish off a meal with an exotic cheese cake which they have remembered to take out of the freezer while they were heating the tinned steak and kidney pudding. To make it all even more attractive, the nutritional value of these foods is unchanged, so you don't have to worry about your state of nutritional health.

The question is, can we afford it? Can the world economy go on supporting the vast cost in resources that is required by manufactured processed food? Take, for example, frozen fruit and vegetables. Nearly one-quarter of the total frozen food industry is devoted to the frozen pea. To accommodate this, pea growers now grow only those breeds of peas which are suitable for processing. The peas must be of uniform size, have long pods on long stalks so that the combine harvester can pick them, all ripen at exactly the same time (to the day), and not lose flavour on freezing. The breeds are thus narrowed down to one or two.

A high yield is essential or they are not worth picking, so artificial fertilizers are used; the crop is picked and podded by machinery and then frozen. After that, they must never be allowed to warm up until they are eaten, which means refrigerated storehouses, refrigerated juggernauts to transport them, refrigerated cabinets in the supermarket, and deep-freeze units in the home. Can we afford all this so that we may eat peas all the year round? (And remember, before the strains available were so limited, the pea season lasted from June through to November, almost half the year.)

Another example is textured vegetable protein (TVP). By great ingenuity, and the expenditure of yet more energy, soy beans can be turned into something that looks like meat. They can then be added to hamburgers, sausages, and meat pies and the consumer is often quite unaware that there are any beans present. Why? What is wrong with beans? The sun will dry them out after harvest, free, gratis, and for nothing. They can then be cooked in a hundred delicious ways, as they have been for centuries in many countries.

These are the questions we have to ask when we wonder about the economy of processed foods. Are we using renewable resources like the sun to dry beans, salt to preserve herrings, bacteria to ferment milk into cheese? Or are we using energy from solid or liquid fuel, thereby depleting the supply in a world which is already worried about the energy crisis? Are we practising wise economy? Or are we guilty of wicked waste?

21 Health foods

In the previous chapter I talked about the nostalgia which has made people want to go backwards in time and eat the good old food of Grandma's day, in the hope that it will make them more healthy. Commercial interests have been quick to exploit this nostalgia, with the result that there is now a wide range of foods available labelled 'health foods', often in packages which look old fashioned, containing food which claims to improve your health. What is a health food? It is a food sold in a health-food shop. What is a health-food shop? A shop which sells health foods! Our language has acquired a phrase for which there seems to be no specific meaning.

Do health foods make you healthy? Let's compare some of the most popular members of this group of foods with their corresponding 'non-health' partners.

Wholegrain cereal This includes wholemeal (wholewheat, high-extraction) flour, wholegrain (brown) rice, and whole oats. These wholegrains contain more of the outer husk and the germ of the grain than do milled varieties. They therefore contain more fibre and more B-group vitamins and slightly more protein. Their advantages are discussed more fully on page 43 but, briefly, their nutritional advantage is related to their high fibre content. This facilitates emptying of the bowel and may confer other benefits as well.

Strong white flour Some wheats, generally grown in drier climates (U.S.A. and Canada), are called hard wheats; they contain a high percentage of the protein, gluten. Most wheat grown in the U.K. is soft wheat and contains less gluten. Gluten is sticky and helps maintain the shape of the loaf when bread rises. Strong white flour is made from hard wheat (high gluten); it may produce a better shaped loaf, but it has no nutritional advantage over ordinary white flour.

Peas, beans, lentils, and nuts These foods are all seeds and contain a large quantity of protein, about one-fifth of the dry weight being protein compared to one-eighth in wheat. The protein is short of the essential amino acids which contain sulphur (meat tends to be low in the same amino acids). Wheat, on the other hand, contains adequate quantities of these sulphur-containing amino acids but is short of another amino acid, lysine, which is present in high quantities in the pulses. Wheat and pulses therefore complement each other in providing a full range of essential amino acids, and for the vegetarian the pulses are a valuable source of protein. For the non-vegetarian they make a cheap and tasty alternative to meat.

In addition to protein, pulses are a very good source of the vitamins of the B group. Also, *sprouting* pulses (bean shoots) are very rich in vitamin C; this source may be important if fresh vegetables are not available.

Baked beans in tins may be regarded as the equivalent non-health form of beans and are a very common item of diet in many developed countries. They have the nutritional advantages described above; baked beans on toast is a highly nutritious meal. Their only disadvantage is that they contain sugar. The same applies to peanut butter.

Honey and brown sugar See page 40 but, briefly, they are just as *bad* for you as white sugar. They may contain some minerals (chromium and iron). To eat enough to make this significant would require an excessive intake of sugar.

Yeast (also yeast tablets, yeast extracts such as Marmite and Vegemite, etc.) These are fine for raising bread, or spreading on it, but unnecessary as an extra source of B-group vitamins except in special circumstances (for example, if you are living on polished rice, or in a famine situation).

Wheatgerm This is a rich source of vitamins of the B group and protein which, if you are on a mixed diet, you are already eating in adequate quantities. It is also very rich in vitamin E. The belief that wheatgerm makes you healthy arises from the claim that many diets are deficient in vitamin E. These claims are nonsense: vitamin E deficiency has never been reported in a human.

Cottage cheese and yogurt These are both clotted-milk products, made by adding bacteria to milk. They contain exactly the same nutrients as milk, that is they are a good source of high-value protein and calcium. If they are made from *skimmed* milk (they usually are) the fat has been removed and you are eating solid fatless milk; the equivalent quantities are as follows: 1 measure skimmed milk is equal to 1 measure of yogurt or to half a measure of cottage cheese. Live yogurt is yogurt which still contains the living bacteria which have fermented it. It is therefore useful for making your own yogurt. It has no known nutritional (or digestive) advantage over dead yogurt.

Dried fruits These contain hardly any vitamin C, but some iron. They are over half sugar in its most dangerous (sticky) form for your teeth. Too much of them carries the same dangers as too much sugar. (However, they are delicious. During the war dried bananas were available; they were nothing like fresh bananas, but loved for their own sake. Some people feel the same about sultanas, which are totally lacking in any resemblance to grapes.)

Muesli This breakfast cereal usually contains oats, nuts, sultanas, and various other ingredients. Unfortunately, the various other ingredients often include sugar. Oats are better for you than many modern breakfast cereals (which usually consist of some form of refined carbohydrate, toasted to golden perfection and mixed with plastic toys) because oats contain roughage. The nuts in muesli will give you some protein. The rest of muesli (sugar and sultanas) is there just for the taste. On the whole it would be better to make your own muesli from rolled oats and add some nuts and, if you can't live without them, a few sultanas.

These, then, are a few examples of health foods. Over all, if you buy food in a health shop, your health will be neither worse nor better than if you buy everything at the supermarket. The people who run health-food shops, however, are usually interested in what they sell while the assistants in supermarkets are usually not so. Also, sacks of beans and rice are somehow more attractive than acres of tins and bottles and cardboard packets. The price for non-conformity is always high, so be prepared to pay extra in a health-food shop.

22 How to improve your diet

How do you know whether there is any need to improve your diet? Answer the following five questions:

Are you over 30 years of age?
Are you a low-risk cardiac patient?
Are you the weight you want to be?
Are you in good health?
Are you managing to keep the cost of your food low?

If you answer YES to all these questions, then you are almost certainly eating an adequate diet and not loading it too much with useless foods. Continue to eat as you do at present, and enjoy it!

If, however, you are younger, or looking after young people, or you want to make changes for either health or financial reasons, there is good precedent to do so. The governments of the United States and Great Britain set up committees to examine national diets and make suggestions for change if necessary: the reports were published in 1977 and 1978 respectively. In addition, in 1979 three prominent British nutritionists (Passmore, Hollingsworth, and Robertson) published an article in the *British Medical Journal* called 'Prescription for a Better British Diet'. Every one of these reports suggested that changes in the national diet would improve health, and in most cases the changes suggested were similar. Much of the following summary is drawn from these reports.

The advice is summarized in two sections. The first section is about dietary deficiencies. These exist, even in affluent societies. The four most common ones are listed; work out if you are in any of the groups affected and if you are, take steps to remedy it. Remember, long-term correction of deficiencies is more effectively achieved by improving the diet than by giving supplements in the form of tablets.

Dietary deficiencies in affluent societies

Deficiency	People at risk	What to eat to cure it
Iron (anaemia, resulting in tiredness)	Women who suffer more than average menstrual loss. Women who have had two or more pregnancies in quick succession. Anyone who has lost a lot of blood. Growing children.	The best dietary source of iron is MEAT. Best vegetable sources are green vegetables, eaten together with vitamin C. Tablets may be necessary.
Vitamin C (scurvy, resulting in tiredness and, later, bleeding)	The old. The poor. Those living alone. Busy people eating tinned food.	Eat *two* of the following each day: A piece of fresh fruit. A green vegetable carefully cooked. A serving of potatoes. If you are worried about it, take tablets: 30 mg per day or 1 gram each month.
Calcium and/or vitamin D (poor bones and teeth)	Pregnant women and children in low-income families, especially in low-sunlight countries.	Sunlight is the best way of getting vitamin D; cod-liver oil may be necessary. For calcium, milk and cheese are best; pulses and cereals fair.
Vitamin B_{12} (anaemia, then unco-ordinated movement)	People who are on a very strict vegetarian diet, that is eating no milk, cheese, or eggs as well as no meat, fish, or chicken. The developing baby is especially at risk.	There are no plant sources. While you are pregnant and lactating and if your principles allow it, drink half a litre of milk a day. If not, explain your diet to your doctor; he can test for deficiency and prescribe supplements.

The second section lists six suggestions for better eating, in what I consider order of importance. These make a convenient summary: a sort of 'take-home' message. Because they are in summary form, however, they do unavoidably seem authoritarian. This is not the intention, so while you are reading them remember they are meant only as ADVICE. Do not follow them slavishly if they cut across special preferences; also, details may change as more research is carried out! However, in my opinion this is the best advice available at the present time.

Suggestions to improve your diet

1. *Eat a varied diet* (the most important rule of all and particularly if you are on a special diet)

Base it on potatoes and bread.
Add each day:
    At least one yellow or green vegetable.
    At least one piece of fruit.
    One high-protein food (see page 55).
But within these groups, have at least five varieties each week.

2. *Eat less empty calories* (sugar and alcohol)

Treat them as 'party' food and drink, having them as treats but not regular meals.
(This includes all alcoholic drinks, soft drinks, sweets, biscuits, cakes, and puddings.)

3. *Eat less animal fat* (especially high-risk cardiac patients)

Eat less meat. Cut visible fat off meat.
Replace butter with polyunsaturated margarine.
Cook in polyunsaturated oils.
Don't forget chocolate is nearly half fat!

4. *Eat more potatoes and bread* (especially if you want to save money)

Eat more meatless meals.
Have sandwiches for lunch.
Have more potatoes and less meat at dinner.

5. *Eat more fibre* (especially those trying to lose weight and those with constipation)

Eat wholegrain cereals like wholemeal bread, brown rice, and oats.
Eat more fruit and vegetables.

6. *Eat less salt* (especially babies and children)

Do not add salt to babies' food.
If you are the family cook, add less salt when cooking.
Use the salt sparingly at table.

Bibliography

General (Chapters 1, 5, 6, 7, 9, 10, 11, 22)

For those wishing to read further in the general field of nutrition, I would suggest three books:

Breckon, W. *You Are What You Eat* (BBC Publications, 1976).

Fisher, P. and Bender, A. *The Value of Food* (Oxford University Press, 1979).

Davidson, S., Passmore, R., Brock, J. F., and Trusswell, A. S. *Human Nutrition and Dietetics* (Churchill Livingstone, 1975).

In addition, there are two official publications which are worth reading:

Department of Health and Social Security *Prevention and Health: Eating for Health* (H.M.S.O., London, 1978).

Ministry of Agriculture, Fisheries, and Food *Manual of Nutrition* (H.M.S.O., London, 1978).

Other reading

For those with an interest in specialized areas, the following will suggest other further reading.

Chapters 2 and 3: most diet books are too limited in their approach, many are wrong, and some give advice that is dangerous. Buy instead one of the slimming magazines (e.g. *Slimming*, *Weightwatchers*, *Successful Slimming*, or *Slimming Naturally*). These give you a broad view of what is happening in the slimming world, since they contain articles from many writers, and on the whole give common-sense advice. They also (if you are trying to lose weight) make you feel part of a group of other people with the same aim.

Chapter 4: many of the publications from War on Want (467 Caledonian Road, London N7 9BE) are relevant, particularly *The Baby Killer Scandal* by Andy Chetley (1979). A book which will introduce you to the politics of starvation is *The Famine Business* by Colin Tudge (Faber and Faber, 1977).

Chapter 5: *English Bread and Yeast Cookery* by Elizabeth David (Penguin Books, 1977) is a delightful and informative book. If you are interested in the fibre story, read *Taking the Rough with the Smooth* by A. Stanway (Pan Books, 1976).

Chapter 8: *Alcohol and Alcoholism* (Tavistock Publications, 1979) is a report of a special committee of the Royal College of Psychiatrists. It is written in terms readily understood by the lay person, and has a good list of further suggested reading.

Chapter 12: *The Know-How of Infant Feeding* by Sylvia Close (John Wright, Bristol, 1973).

Chapter 14: *Textbook of Work Physiology* by P.-O. Astrand and K. Rodahl (McGraw-Hill, 1977), Ch. 14. This is a bit on the technical side but athletic coaches will find it rewarding reading.

Chapter 16: *Coronary Heart Disease*, report of a joint working party of the Royal College of Physicians of London and the British Cardiac Society (1976).

Chapter 17: *The Prevention of Food Poisoning* by J. Trickett (Stanley Thornes, 1978).

Index